CARMEN M. PEREZ
The Wellbeing Messenger

BE A
SPIRITUAL GIRL
In a Material World

Achieve Radical Personal Success
Without Sacrificing Your
Health, Wealth, and Happiness

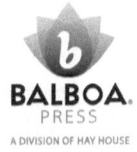

BALBOA.
PRESS
A DIVISION OF HAY HOUSE

Balboa Press books may be ordered through booksellers or by contacting:

Balboa Press
A Division of Hay House
1663 Liberty Drive
Bloomington, IN 47403
www.balboapress.com
1 (877) 407-4847

Because of the dynamic nature of the Internet, any web addresses or
links contained in this book may have changed since publication and
may no longer be valid. The views expressed in this work are solely those
of the author and do not necessarily reflect the views of the publisher,
and the publisher hereby disclaims any responsibility for them.

The author of this book does not dispense medical advice or prescribe the use
of any technique as a form of treatment for physical, emotional, or medical
problems without the advice of a physician, either directly or indirectly. The
intent of the author is only to offer information of a general nature to help
you in your quest for emotional and spiritual well-being. In the event you use
any of the information in this book for yourself, which is your constitutional
right, the author and the publisher assume no responsibility for your actions.

Any people depicted in stock imagery provided by Thinkstock are models,
and such images are being used for illustrative purposes only.
Certain stock imagery © Thinkstock.

Print information available on the last page.

ISBN: 978-1-5043-9308-9 (sc)
ISBN: 978-1-5043-9310-2 (hc)
ISBN: 978-1-5043-9309-6 (e)

Library of Congress Control Number: 2017918688

Balboa Press rev. date: 01/26/2018

Be a Spiritual Girl in a Material World
By Carmen M. Perez, The Wellbeing Messenger

Achieve Radical Personal Success Without Sacrificing
Your Health, Wealth, and Happiness

PRAISE FOR
BE A SPIRITUAL GIRL IN A
MATERIAL WORLD

I consider myself an intelligent, motivated entrepreneur but began feeling overwhelmed with trying to please everyone in my business and personal life, and frustrated that I was not accomplishing the day-to-day items that needed to be taken care of. I spent time reading and studying from many sources but felt paralyzed with the many great ideas but no real plan to put any of them in place.

Then I began reading Carmen Perez's *Be a Spiritual Girl in a Material World*. As early as the Introduction, I thought, "Wow! This is Awesome!" It was as if Carmen was speaking to me personally and yet I couldn't wait to share it as I saw how it could benefit family and friends who were in very different stages of life. I like that Carmen has taken what she learned from the struggles in her life, along with the struggles of those she has coached, to develop a simple yet powerfully effective step-by-step approach to make the changes needed to improve not only your business but your overall quality of life.

Carmen's book is a real life-changer. Exercises throughout each chapter guided me through the process necessary to get beyond the chaos and move to the next step. The processes used for finding our top, workable, thriving goals in business and all areas of our life, as well as Carmen's Top 10 Lists for Effective Productivity, became tremendous time savers and helped me shift from one task to the next without wasting precious time trying to figure out what to do next.

~Jeanine Fey

Before reading Carmen's book, *Be a Spiritual Girl in a Material World*, I felt unworthy, overwhelmed, and a little on the chaotic side. As I read, I started feeling more and more at peace. I felt like I had a friend who had been through things I'm going through and worse, and that she understood, and did so in an uncondescending way.

Carmen's guidance, advice, and wisdom helped me feel worthy, peaceful and very grateful. The strategies that she shares to have a more fulfilling, purposeful life are a godsend. My favorite things in the book are the different lists to help keep me more organized!

This book will stay on my shelf in the reference section as I know I'll refer back to it many times when I need a quick pick-me-up and a reminder of my value. Thank you, Carmen, for shining your light so brightly in this beautiful book.

~Shannon Cunningham LeBlanc

As a mom, woman, and entrepreneur I have struggled with juggling too many plates. I can really take the wind out of me some days. I can get to the point of throwing in the towel. I get overwhelmed knowing I have so much to do and don't know where to start or how to get to where I want to go. It is emotionally and mentally draining at times.

Reading *Be a Spiritual Girl in a Material World* gave me a road map and plan to help me change how I approached the overwhelm and frustration in my life. I found steps to help center myself, as well as a reminder that I don't have to do it all today. I can take time for me. My Flight Plan helped me weed through all the muck I put on myself and now I know where I am going.

I was touched by Carmen's sharing of her journey and path. There were many places where I was like YES that's me. I feel the same way. I am not alone. I was struck will all that she had gone through and took back her health and her life. That she has set boundaries for time to care for her and her journey. I don't have to feel guilty to do the same.

The Spiritual Prescriptions were easy to follow, as well as the steps that I can take to move forward in my own life. I got real, practical tips and steps to work and do, which I really liked. I am a practical girl, so I like being offered activities and tools that I can use in my own journey.

Carmen comes from a real place of wanting to be a light for others. I felt that in reading *Be a Spiritual Girl*. I felt how genuine she is in what she shares. I was able to connect with her and her journey, which made me feel at ease in what I need to do and where I need to go. I took away a sense of peace and real tools and steps that I can weave into my own life and journey.

~Kim Milnes

If I had to be honest, I didn't think I was in a place that I "needed" Be a Spiritual Girl in a Material World. BOY OH BOY was I in for a rude awakening! My initial intention was to just read the book, not USE the book. After all, me and my life were just fine! But I very quickly realized that I couldn't read it without thinking about and applying this to my life. I had no idea how disconnected I was until I read it; moments in the book actually stole my breath because they were such AH-HA moments.

One of the things that made this all possible was that it really just felt like we were sitting down having a conversation between friends . . . like Carmen knew what I needed and where I was coming from. Reading this book has released me from some emotions that I didn't even realize I was holding onto.

I had chosen to forget that I can't expect people to be what I want them to be, or to give back what I give to them (emotionally); in all of that I had the guidance to not hold it against myself or them for what I hoped for them to be. My biggest AH-HA moment was the permission to let go of things that no longer serve me, even relationships that I may feel very vested in. Before this book, I held on, even though at times I was miserable. I mean, if I quit it would feel like giving up. Since then, I have let go of many things that were toxic in my life and no longer serve me and I'm fine . . . better than fine, I feel like a weight has been lifted!

My favorite AH-HA moment was happitunities. I hadn't thought of it like that. I NEED THAT! I instantly thought of 50 people who need that! Such a great way to think and be! I firmly believe this book is going to change so many lives, even for those who may not think they need it!

~Jenny Sennett

I have struggled for many years with work/personal life balance. I felt overwhelmed, frustrated and literally made myself sick by working too much. Although I have a successful business, I was not loving my job and felt like quitting many times. I could easily relate to Carmen's book as her story sounded much like mine.

Carmen clearly explains each element of The Flight Plan as a guide to live a life of wellbeing. Balance is still a work in progress, but with The Flight Plan, I am learning to take control of my days. In particular, the section on Effective Productivity with its step-by-step instructions and examples on Creating a Daily Agenda was very helpful. If you need guidance for a lifestyle change, I highly recommend that you read *Be a Spiritual Girl in a Material World*.

~Kathy Takushi

As a busy professional, I am faced with multiple, high-priority demands on my attention and energy on a daily basis. I've often felt overwhelmed when looking at my to-do list, wondering how I'll possibly get everything done, let alone, done well. I also understand the importance of balancing work with my spiritual practice, so I was immediately drawn to Carmen's book, which is filled with practical wisdom from someone who can relate.

I was really moved by Carmen's honesty and vulnerability in sharing her story. And her Flight Plan system is a lifeline to help busy women like me stay organized, grounded, and sane.

Thank you, Carmen, for creating such a helpful resource for those of us who seek to create a successful, heart-centered business and life!

~Christine Love

I have felt alone in the Material World most of my life, as if I was an outsider watching life happen. I felt I had no control over my life. I have wanted to feel like I belonged my entire life. I was abandoned by my parents when I was 7 and never got out of the child foster system until I was eighteen. I don't know why I was put here to go through the things I have gone through, but *Be a Spiritual Girl in a Material World*, has given me hope and faith that I am here for a reason and good things are going to happen in my life.

The book helped me understand that I do not have to keep living silently as a bystander. I feel like Carmen has given me the permission I needed and waited for my entire life, to live out loud and let people see me.

The Flight Plan has helped me find my purpose and I am so excited about my future, more than I have ever been. The Spiritual Prescriptions helped me define what I want my life to mean. I have been through a lot and now I know I am not alone, and I can do and have everything that I want.

I have enrolled in night school. I don't know what I want to do yet, but I know I'll discover it there.

Carmen, thank you for writing this book for me, and people like me.

~Elle McCarthy

Be a Spiritual Girl
in a Material World

To my family, Fred, Migdalia, Roque, and Reyna.
You are my reason for everything.

ACKNOWLEDGMENTS

Countless people have influenced me and, hence, played a part in the creation of this book. Please know the words that follow are only a small portion of the boundless gratitude I feel for your contribution, presence, and support of my life and this book.

To my family and friends, you know in your heart who you are: Thank you for accepting me for who I am and cheering me on as I discover my purpose without judgment. I don't know where I would be or who I would be without you. I was lost, and because of your support, I am found. You have inspired me and given me permission to connect to my true self.

To inspiring influencers and mentors Brendon Burchard, Marianne Williamson, Gabrielle Bernstein, Nick Ortner, Deepak Chopra, Steven Covey, Oprah Winfrey, Carolyn Myss, the late Dr. Wayne Dyer and Louise Hay: Thank you for shining your light and giving me and everyone else permission to shine ours. Because of your work, I found my true self and tapped into my true potential. Some of you have personally given me the guidance I needed, and some have given in absentia. Either way, know it has made an impact for which I will be forever grateful.

To my team at Wellbeing Messenger: Thank you for your dedication and willingness to give your all so we can make a difference in the world. It is an honor and privilege to be on this journey with you.

To Meredith Hill and Vanessa McGovern: I am deeply appreciative of finding you when I needed you most. To say that you are soul sisters is an understatement. You are cheerleaders, dream facilitators, and teachers, and I thank you for your inspiration to write this book.

To Gina Hogan Edwards: I am grateful for your encouragement, guidance, and expertise helped me articulate what is in my heart so I could share it in this book.

To my clients and students of Wellbeing Messenger and Get Noticed Online Now: Thank you for consistently demanding I show up as the best and highest version of myself, with authenticity, gratitude, integrity, and love. This book would not be possible without you.

To Misty: Thank you for being the perfect little sister who annoyed me in all the right ways and gave me three perfect little nieces to love. I am so proud of you and the woman you are.

To Mom and Mando: I am grateful for your love, support, strength, and courage.

To Margie: Thank you for being the first light I saw when I was lost during those teen years. I appreciate you and am so grateful for your love and support at a very dark and lonely time.

To Natalie Cindy: Thank you for being my best friend, and co-conspirator. You helped me discover the person I had the potential to be. Your unconditional love during the last three decades has given me strength and courage to discover my path.

To my grandchildren Avriel and Amaya: Thank you for being perfect in every way: Know I will always support and love you unconditionally and without judgment.

To my children Migdalia, Roque, and Reyna: Thank you for being constant reminders of why I needed to discover how to create a life worth living.

To my husband Fred: Thank you for accepting and loving all the versions of me, unconditionally. There are no words that would ever fully acknowledge the depth of what your love and support in my life means to me. I admire you. I respect you. I honor you, and I love you with all my heart and soul.

CONTENTS

Praise For Be A Spiritual Girl In A Material World vii

Acknowledgments xv

Foreword... xxi

A Personal Note xxiii

Introduction.. xxvii

Section 1: Where are you now? 1

    Chapter 1 Survive by Default................................ 3

    Chapter 2 Thrive by Design 31

Section 2: Where do you want to go? 53

    Chapter 3 The Flight Plan................................. 55

        Spiritual Prescription for Clarity............................ 70

    Chapter 4 Live with Passion 71

        Principle 1 of a Thriving Mindset | Be Mindfully Aware.... 80

        Spiritual Prescription for Mindful Awareness 86

        Principle 2 of a Thriving Mindset | Be Willing 88

        Spiritual Prescription for Willingness 94

        Principle 3 of a Thriving Mindset | Be Committed........ 98

        Spiritual Prescription for Commitment 123

    Chapter 5 Live with Purpose............................. 125

        Spiritual Prescription for Direction....................... 132

    Calm the CHAOS ~ Connection 134

        Spiritual Prescription for Meaningful Connections ... 158

    Calm the CHAOS ~ Health and Wellness.................. 161

Spiritual Prescription for Health and Wellness 170
Calm the CHAOS ~ Achievement............................ 173
    Spiritual Prescription to Make Your Dreams
    Your Reality 182
Calm the CHAOS ~ Organization 186
    Spiritual Prescription to Set Yourself Up for
    Success 191
Calm the CHAOS ~ Spirituality 193
    Spiritual Prescription for Spirituality 204
Chapter 6 Live with Play... 207
    Spiritual Prescription for Living in Alignment....... 220
    Key 1 | Thoughtfulness... 225
    Key 2 | Regulate 229
    Key 3 | Assign... 235
    Key 4 | Vigilance 246
    Key 5 | Extract.. 249
    Key 6 | Learn.. 255
    Key 7 | Self-Love.. 257
    The Secret Key.. 264

Section 3: Are you ready to thrive? 273
Chapter 7 Commit to a Life Worth Living......................... 275

Meet the Author... 285

FOREWORD

We live in an extraordinary time in human history. Technological advancements allow us to be more connected than at any other time in human history. Communication tools connect us at lightning speeds, which has created a culture that thrives on instant gratification and material-driven desires. This way of living has yielded growth and abundance in the external world, but, ironically, this intensity of growth is leaving us increasingly disconnected from one another and, most importantly, from our souls. *Be a Spiritual Girl in a Material World* is not a book that teaches a new way of living in a material world, but rather, it is a book that creates the space for you to return to your authentic self and your natural-born ambitions and desires.

We have lost ourselves in our fast-paced, material-focused world. Our lifestyles leave us craving more joy, more happiness, and more meaningful connections. Distractions in our day are endless, and living a simple and effortless life often seems unachievable.

Carmen Perez is a lighthouse amidst all the digital and material chaos, and she is shining her light to illuminate a path that can empower us to transform how we experience the world. She brings balance and practical insights to how we process the noise that bombards us every day. Carmen's Spiritual Prescriptions are our remedy to thrive and tap into the magical beauty of life. If we all unite to implement what Carmen outlines in this book, we will unquestionably raise the vibrations on our planet and influence the next generation of women to experience life more soulfully and in line with their true purpose.

Carmen's book is a gift to women and is timely for what we are emotionally craving. Get ready to experience amazing shifts and gain access to executable strategies for redefining your experiences so you can live a more abundant and amplified life.

Vanessa McGovern

Co-Founder and CEO of Gifted Travel Network

Wife, mother of two, Japanese Chin lover, and travel industry advocate

A PERSONAL NOTE

As an author, high-performance coach, master practitioner of the Law of Attraction, certified Neurolinguistics Programming Practitioner, motivational speaker, wellbeing and travel expert, and personal business success mentor, I have been incredibly blessed to work with phenomenal heart-centered, purpose-driven, soulful businesses and entrepreneurs. What I share with you in this book is my perspective of my experiences and efforts to create a life worth living.

I share things I have learned through mentors and have personally experienced in my life; things I have learned and practiced while supporting my family, friends, clients, fans, and audiences, who were struggling and feeling stuck in a world filled with promise that they were unable to connect with; and things I have learned from doctors and fellow patients, fighting to calm the chaos so lives could be saved. I share what I have discovered to create a life worth living when mine was not.

I share these things so you can create a life in which you experience bliss more often and bitterness much less; a life in which you feel loved and never insignificant, valued and never unworthy of good fortune, heard and never ignored, respected and never neglected, empowered and never powerless, and a life in which you overcome fear.

I am not a doctor, psychologist, psychotherapist, psychiatrist, or nutritionist. I am a student of life, much like you. I firmly believe that my experiences have been what they have been and my life was spared so I could share what I have learned to calm the chaos in the Material World. I help people connect with their ability, clarity, creativity, inspiration, and talent to achieve the success they desire without sacrificing their health, wealth, and happiness.

None of the information I share with you is meant to be medical, legal, or professional advice. I share the things that have empowered me and thousands of women all over the world so you can be empowered too.

My intention is to awaken you. Awaken you to stop living by default and start living by design. Awaken you to heal what ails your soul and makes your heart ache. Awaken you to invite the joy you desire into your life. Awaken you to the fact that you are here to thrive and surviving should not be the default for a well-lived life.

If you need professional help, I implore you to find it. Reach out to a confidant, or talk to your doctor.

If you are curious and want to dig into a topic further, I encourage you to do so. Do research, read books, search Google. There is a wealth of information out there for you.

If you have questions about my work, please reach out to me at WMOffice@WellbeingMessenger.com. I am here to be of service to you. For additional resources, visit my book website, www. BeASpiritualGirl.com.

The message of my book is to create a life worth living that serves your greatest and highest good, which allows you to realize your full, desired potential. You alone create your health, wealth, and happiness. This book will empower you to build a life worth living by calming the chaos of this Material World. I am honored to serve as your guide. I cannot wait to celebrate your transformation with you.

With so much love and gratitude,

Carmen M. Perez, Your Wellbeing Messenger

INTRODUCTION

"The real voyage of discovery consists not in seeking new landscapes, but in having new eyes." -Marcel Proust

How is it that today, when we can have and be anything we want, we do not choose to be happy?

Instead, we choose to do things for what they get us, not for what they do for us. Instead, we choose to work in careers that do not feed our hunger for purpose. Instead, we choose to say "Yes" even when we should say "No." Instead, we choose to live by default, accepting whatever life throws at us. Instead, we choose to do the things we think we should be doing even when they do not feel good. Instead, we wrestle against the current, fighting our way through, holding the hope that, eventually, we will get our just rewards—in retirement, if we are lucky, or heaven, perhaps, if that's what it takes.

We allow our stress to control our emotions and to dictate the level of success we can achieve. We have handed over our personal power to the discretion and influence of the chaos, mass media, and reality television. Because of it, our health is suffering. We numb ourselves with liquor, pills, or other addictive behaviors that blur the lines of our chosen path, instead of healing our lives with love, fulfillment, and meaning. We harshly judge those who are lost and cannot seem to find their way, rather than offering a helping hand. We are the ones making this a chaotic Material World. However, all is not lost. Seven percent (7%) of the population has figured it out.

The 7% who have conditioned their mindset understand how to generate love, fulfillment, and meaning in their lives. They have achieved health, wealth, and happiness. They invest the time to make an impact on the quality of their lives. They have mastered fulfilling connections, health and wellness, achievement, organization, and spirituality.

The Material World

The Material World is our "reality," which is often depicted as chaotic, noisy, and unforgiving. This "reality" lures us in with a depiction of success that comes at the cost of our mortality and wellbeing. We watch chaotic lives that reward hard work with unfulfilled desires and stress and that laugh at those who live with passion, purpose, and play. This "reality" prevents most from stepping out and deciding to thrive, when surviving has become the norm.

Until my discoveries, life always felt so hard, as if I had to earn happiness. I learned that there is hope and a simple way to live from an inspired place. By reclaiming our time and focusing on what matters, we can transform the way we experience the Material World, empowering us to create thriving lives filled with connection, courage, and compassion. Today, I have a unique understanding of the difficulties in recommitting to hope and personal wellbeing, and I believe it will empower you to transform the way you experience your Material World.

I have seen the doctors. I have read the books. And I have lived the chaos and time famines. I have discovered how to be more Spiritual in a Material World so YOU can create the life you have always dreamed of but, for some reason, have been unable to fully commit to creating.

You do not have to lose everything to get there or hit rock bottom like I, and too many others, did. You can start right now by awakening and committing to your desire to create a life worth living.

Be a Spiritual Girl

Being a Spiritual Girl in a Material World means you think differently than the norm. You create a life you love without apology, compromise, or guilt. You focus on what matters to calm the chaos of the Material World. You clearly know what you want and see the path to achieve it. You know how to move confidently in the direction of your dreams. You allow yourself to feel and show gratitude for what you have and experience. You choose to love more and fear less. You know what you need to do and do it when you say you are going to do it. You proactively and progressively close the gap between where you are and where you want to be. You feel empowered to overcome the challenges that arise. You step fully into your light and brilliance to create a life worth living by your terms.

Within the pages of this book, I share my experience, knowledge, and strategies, created, learned, and practiced, to achieve and maintain my wellbeing so that you can too. I am sharing what I have learned because I believe we are all here to thrive.

I am not just going to share what to do. I am going to share with you, step by step, how to do it, so that you can live with passion, purpose, and play.

Use this book as a guide to attain the personal success you have always desired without sacrificing your health, wealth, and happiness.

I promise to keep it simple, but impactful. Know that what you want is achievable and that creating a life worth living will empower you to make your dreams your reality.

Spiritual Girl's Medicine Chest | Spiritual Prescriptions

I created the Spiritual Prescriptions you'll find throughout this book as a way for us to clean up years of sloppy thinking that have caused dis-ease, dysfunction, and discomfort in our lives. They will help you do away with the chaos and toxic habits to bring the effortlessness you crave and deserve.

The Spiritual Prescriptions fill the Spiritual Girl's Medicine Chest. They are processes and strategies to help you achieve and maintain a sense of ease and flow in your life. You can do them anywhere, anytime. They are deliberately simple so you can use them whenever things come up, no matter where you are. As you apply each Spiritual Prescription, you fill your Spiritual Girl's Medicine Chest. This is how you reclaim your power to create a life worth living defined by you and for you.

Each prescription is an antidote for what ails your soul and your life. When you feel you have fallen off your path and are out of alignment, look to your Spiritual Prescriptions.

I honor you for doing this work. This is the tough work. This is the work that causes true transformation in your character and, hence, transcendence.

Section 1

WHERE ARE YOU NOW?

To move forward in life, we must look at where we are now. We must understand:

The experiences we have had.

The choices we have made.

The dreams we have left behind.

This is our journey and understanding where we are now allows us to embrace the process of creating a life worth living.

In Chapter 1, you will see how living by default in the Material World has fueled the acceptance of mere survival.

In Chapter 2, you will see how to thrive by designing your life so it leads to fulfillment, meaning, and total wellbeing.

Chapter 1

Survive by Default

"Stop looking for the path of least resistance.
Start looking for your next big adventure."
Don't go for easy. Go for ease.
Don't go for now. Go for joy.
Don't go for fear. Go for love."
~Carmen M. Perez

It's Friday, February 11, 2011. My hands are bloody and filled with my hair. I curl up on the bathroom floor in tears. My mobile phone is next to me. Through my tears, I make out the time: 11:11 a.m. I'm done. I'm sick and tired of being sick and tired. I am lost, and I do not know what to do.

I lie there on that floor after giving every ounce of my energy to a fit of rage because of The Illness, with a capital "I." The Illness had left me bedridden for nearly a year. It had me certain that my days were numbered and that by the time we found out what it was, I would be dead. I'm on this floor because of another disappointing call from my doctor.

With nothing left in me, I sleep for the better part of two days, crying and praying I will not wake up. I have no more fight.

Then came a radical shift, a miracle.

When Sunday morning arrived, I was ready. I made a commitment. I made the promise to myself that I was going to stop surviving and start thriving. I was no longer willing to accept my circumstances. I would find another way, a different way, a better-feeling way, to create a life worth living. I refused to let this be my end.

I made this fateful day my beginning.

On this day, I, Carmen Michelle Perez, do hereby solemnly swear to accept the challenge to achieve success by living with passion, purpose, and play, and to never compromise my health, wealth, and happiness.

I refer to this time in my life as "The Illness." Using this term gives me some distance from it; I no longer own this condition.

* * *

Imagine living in complete joy and feeling more ease in your day-to-day life. Imagine:

> Living each day focused on the things that matter to you most; Taking action when necessary and, just like magic, the Universe conspires on your behalf to deliver exactly what you ask; and
> Going through your days feeling good and in total control of your health, wealth, and happiness.

Wouldn't it be nice if life worked this way?

However, most of us are, at best, content taking what comes our way, feeling like life is hard and the Material World is working against us. We survive the day-to-day humdrum without inspiration or purpose, feeling as though we have no control or responsibility for our quality of life, hoping that—if we're lucky—we might end up somewhere we like being.

Wellbeing

Do you ever feel empty inside when everything
on the outside seems complete and joyful?

It is not uncommon to feel bad even when things outside look, well, pretty good. As we do the things we are told are all the "right" things and look good to everybody else, we somehow end up drained of our energy and feel unfulfilled.

I don't believe that health is working 50+ hours a week to prove our worth, using money and material things to prove our significance, or pushing ourselves to achieve more power to prove our value to the world. These things have done nothing but make us complacent, simply doing our time, counting the days as we blithely survive from one day to the next.

When feeling run down or burnt out, most people accept this state of being as the way it's supposed to be. They complain but do nothing to change their circumstances. They pop some pills to cope. A small, motivated group will start eating better and/or exercising. But that's not enough. We must not ignore our wellbeing.

Wellbeing is the state of health, wealth, and happiness. To attain a well physical and mental condition is the state of health. To achieve success through meaning and fulfillment is the state of wealth. To have positive and pleasant emotions ranging from contentment to intense joy is the state of happiness. To create a life worth living, we must find new and innovative ways to invest our time, to understand how we want to impact the world, and to live out our deepest desires.

"Health is a state of complete physical, mental and social well-being, and not merely the absence of disease or infirmity." ~World Health Organization

Wellness v. Wellbeing

The terms *wellness* and *wellbeing* often are used interchangeably, but there is a distinctive difference.

Wellbeing refers to a holistic, whole-of-life experience, whereas *wellness* refers specifically to physical health. Wellbeing is a better-than-satisfactory condition of existence, a state characterized by health, happiness, and prosperity.

The Elements of Total Wellbeing

Inherently, we crave five types of wellness in our lives; together, they help us achieve total wellbeing and make life feel more worthwhile. These are the Elements of Total Wellbeing:

Connective Wellness | Creating and maintaining strong relationships and love in your life.

Health Wellness | Having good mental and physical health and enough energy to get things done on a daily basis.

Achievement Wellness | Occupying your time in a way that is satisfying and makes each day feel enjoyable and productive.

Organizational Wellness | Effectively managing your life.

Spiritual Wellness | Connecting to the deepest values and meanings by which you want to live.

My goals for this book are to raise awareness of the devastating side effects of neglecting our wellbeing when we live in the Material World without passion, purpose, and play; and to increase the world's wellbeing by empowering others to live to their highest desired potential. I say "highest desired potential" because our culture pressures us to do what we are good at, not necessarily what we enjoy.

It is time to radically shift our perception of living a life well-lived. It is not enough for me alone to create the love and joy I have always wanted to experience in my life; we must *all* find our health, wealth, and happiness to make this Material World a better place. Otherwise, what's the point of our existence?

What Will Never Change

We will always feel the pull into the drama of others, especially from those we care for and love. That's the fascinating part of the human experience. How you respond to the drama makes all the difference between surviving and thriving. It is your choice whether to live a life in which you feel fully engaged, enlightened, and enthusiastic or overwhelmed, exhausted, and stressed out.

Life Stops for No One

The better we care for our wellbeing, the more empowered we are to respond to life's inevitable throes in a way that honors the essence of who we truly are. Too often, we react in rage by taking out our anger, fear, and resentment on those we love most. And we do it in such a way that we lose out and get further away from what we actually want.

You are here, seeking. Aware that something is not working. Reading this book. Focused. Willing to do things differently and committed to creating a life worth living by your terms. You are no longer living your life by default, accepting what comes to you without considering what will serve your higher personal interests. Feel your way to living the life your soul intended.

Oneness

We don't live in a bubble. We are all one, and for all the things that make us different, there are more things that make us the same. If we all live to our best and highest potential, don't you think it would have an amazing, transcending effect on the Material World, on our life experience? I believe it would, and I would be so honored if you would help me make this dream a reality. Most of us have no vision for what this looks like in our day-to-day lives. Our lack of vision blinds us, and our chaotic environments numb us.

I promise, if you stay with me, you will be empowered to create a life worth living. Transform the way you experience your Material World, calm the chaos, and go from surviving to thriving. We must create a new vision for how we want to live and what we want to experience from a place of knowing how we want to FEEL.

Survival

Common thinking states that the accumulation of our life experiences dictates what we can and cannot achieve. As a society, we have unrealistic expectations of ourselves and others, and we persistently raise the bar. Thus, our happiness levels have steadily declined. We have forgotten why we are here, and we don't live with purpose or on purpose to serve our greatest good. We go for what feels good right now, not for what will feel right a decade from now. We go for short-term gains instead of long-term growth.

It is time to ask ourselves why and to stop ignoring all the signs telling us it's not okay to keep living in this defaulted way.

We look to our economic status, and material possessions to fill us with significance, meaning, and hope. Any lack is an inconvenient reminder of what we dare to desire but do not have the courage to create. Some discover too late—some not at all—that we cannot *find* significance, hope, or anything else worth experiencing. We must *create* those experiences for ourselves.

When we dream, our family tells us, "Be careful, you may get what you ask for," as if that's a bad thing. Our friends say, "You're crazy to think, just because you want it all, that you can have it all," as if wanting it all is wrong. We get messages from watching television and other media, repeatedly showing us that life is supposed to be hard and that surviving another day is our destiny. Thriving doesn't even feel like a choice.

We stop believing in ourselves and forget our commitment to do more than just exist. We turn our backs on our dreams, because we think that what we want is too hard to get or that it's too late or that we've made too many mistakes. We stop trusting in the process of living and enjoying the challenges we encounter in life. We stop connecting to what we truly want. Then, we stop dreaming and do not give ourselves permission to step outside the box people have built for us, and we end up living with regrets, never feeling fulfilled.

We must stop believing we are limited in our abilities and our capacities to achieve what we deeply desire. We are here to experience everything.

The good, the bad, and the ugly are all part of the human experience. Every experience is meant to teach us something. Life is our classroom.

Life is unfair. So what.
Life is hard. So what.
What do these things mean?

Those who ignore the significance of the challenges and the struggles they experience are the ones who have no options and are left feeling stuck. But those who embrace the challenges and honor the struggles are those who create a life worth living.

Let's Talk

No one tells us what we need to know to thrive. They tell us to wear this, buy that, go here, do that. But they don't talk about the important stuff, like those things that help us understand the value of creating a life worth living.

I would like to change that conversation.

Let's talk about creating a life worth living by your terms, your strengths, your preferences, and your likes. Let's talk of the fear and anger that holds us back. Let's talk about the hurts and what keeps us from enjoying life to its fullest. Let's talk about forgiveness, letting go, dealing with guilt, having compassion, and courage. Let's talk of the things that make us human and life more expansive, exciting, and enjoyable. Let's talk about the difference between being alive and living. Let's talk about creating a life that feels good in every way and about being enthused about our days. Let's talk about doing the things that fulfill us and give our lives meaning.

Life is not a punishment. It is a gift—a beautiful, fascinating gift. The challenges, high and low, are all part of it. The ability to feel the emotions that go along with the challenges are part of the adventure. It is not a bad thing to feel anger, outrage, resentment, or any other emotion you may experience. Embrace them all. They provide valuable feedback. Appreciate and give gratitude for each and every one of them. Your ability to experience them means you are not just alive. Rather, you are LIVING.

Invest Your Time

It is important you understand and accept that time is impossible to manage. You get the same amount everyone else gets. There are 24 hours in a day, 60 minutes in an hour, and 60 seconds in a minute—the same for everyone. We cannot manage time. Consider Bill Gates, Mark Zuckerberg, Oprah Winfrey, Elon Musk, Sir Richard Branson, or any other successful person. They don't try to control or manipulate time, yet they are achieving extraordinary things. So, stop trying to manage your time, and, instead, manage your energy and effectiveness.

If you look at your day-to-day actions, what are you doing to close the gap between where you are and where you want to be? What are you doing that feels right and good? I'm not talking about superficial, short-term gains or rewards, such as going out for drinks after a hard day or treating yourself to a brownie when you're feeling stressed. I'm talking about doing the things that will impact your long-term health, wealth, and happiness.

Are you doing things that fulfill you?
Are you connecting to and with the
people you care about most?
Are you generating joy and vitality daily?

Those who understand the value of their time live more deliberately and invest their time wisely. Make no mistake, my friend, it is an investment. Time is a commodity. The more you invest it, the more valuable it is. You cannot buy extra time. There is no shelf at your local big-box store filled with spare minutes. However, most people don't understand the value of their time, and they give it away freely or, worse, they squander it.

We kill time.
We waste time, and we watch time go by.
It's madness and it's time to stop.

The 24-Hour Woman

When I was a little girl in the late 1970s, an Enjoli Perfume commercial played on the television. The woman in the commercial was a beautiful blond. She looked lovely and sparkly. She seemed incredibly happy as she did it all—at least, "all" from my definition at that time. No woman in my life looked like her.

As a ten-year-old girl, I was immediately pulled in. The commercial started with her holding a frying pan and singing, "I can put the wash on the line, feed the kids." In the next scene, in a button-down jacket and pencil skirt with high-heels, pinned up hair, and a purse in hand, she sings, "Get dressed, pass out the kisses, and get to work by five till nine." After the announcer shares, "Enjoli is the eight-hour perfume for the 24-hour woman," we again see the woman in her business look, holding a wad of cash. She sings, "I can bring home the bacon, fry it up in a pan." Then we see her in an evening gown, dressed to the nines and singing, "And never, never, never let you forget you're the man, 'cause I'm a woman. Enjoli."

In my ten-year-old head, everything the perfume commercial represented was entirely possible. For me, that became the epitome of success. Bringing home the bacon, taking care of my home, my family, my man, and looking great while doing it: "The 24-Hour Woman."

This image of the ideal woman that I so desperately wanted to be fiercely maintained its hold on my heart and soul. As I grew up, I became obsessed with how the 24-Hour Woman's life "should" appear. I played the role. Never did I ask, "Is this what I really want my life to look like?"

It was no accident I felt these things about the Enjoli woman. The marketing geniuses for Enjoli wanted precisely that. During the 1960s and 1970s, the media reflected the changes taking place in women's lives. Women were portrayed as having more substantial lives outside the home. Fragrance companies experienced phenomenal growth from the major social changes taking place due to the Women's Movement and the sexual revolution.

When I was 10, all I could think was, "This is the woman I want to be: the 24-Hour Woman." Mrs. Enjoli appeared to have it all. Things seemed so easy for her. She was graceful and her life was so pretty. I fully and completely fell into the illusion. This message was utterly contrary to what I saw in my life. I was being raised by a single, working mother on the northwest side of Chicago, Illinois. There was no grace or effortlessness. Life seemed hard and messy.

By my mid-twenties, I became fixated not only on having it all, but on doing it all. I valued my ability not only to meet, but to surpass expectations. I was prideful of my capacity to work well over 40 hours a week, maintain a clean home, take care of the laundry and shopping, cook the majority of our daily meals, and entertain and party with friends on Friday night. I could spend Saturday with the kids, host dinner at my house that evening, then "relax" Sunday while enjoying the brunch I made, followed by shopping for the week, preparing a traditional Sunday evening dinner, watching a movie with the family, and, finally, getting to bed to do it all over again the following week.

In a study called "The Paradox of Declining Female Happiness," researchers looked into the lives of women in the United States. While they found a significant improvement over the last 40 years, they also showed that women's happiness levels have declined steadily since the Women's Movement, and they are moving in a downward trend, along with men's. When we allow outside influences to set the standards for how we live instead of trusting our inner guidance, we do not feel fulfilled.

Women's freedoms, both in the family and in the marketplace, have grown. Women have gained bargaining power as we make more money. A shift in happiness toward women and away from men was expected. However, men have been the surprise beneficiaries of the Women's Movement. We have indeed increased our power, opportunities, and sexual freedom, all amazing and beautiful things. But we must look at how we have used this power.

Along with the many wonderful benefits of the Women's Movement, we also have increased workloads and manage multiple domains— our homes and the office. While the day-to-day lives of women have substantially changed, expectations around the household have not. The home has become this continually made-over, beautified symbol of status. Women have yet to release the emotional responsibility of their homes and family. As a result, housework has become their second job and our lives are much more complicated.

When men "help" around the house or take care of the children, they are acknowledged for what great husbands and fathers they are. But women are expected to do these things. There is no special recognition. In fact, as mothers, that's not enough. Our children must get good grades, be good, and look good. Our homes must be immaculate, and we must create time to volunteer and entertain. The expectations and judgments are never-ending.

> *Sixty percent (60%) of women are the primary or co-breadwinner but still do most of the housework, according to the Bureau of Labor Statistics.*

The opportunities afforded by the Women's Movement have led to stigmas for women who want to stay home and those who work outside the home. And society judges both. We have to remember either is a good choice; neither is right nor wrong. The choice, though, for many women is actually meaningless because their salaries have become necessary.

When it comes to being a career woman without kids, a working mom, or a stay-at-home mom, we must support one another in our choices. Each requires labor, energy, and dedication. Choose the one that feels right to you and embrace it. There must not be shame or judgment. Some people are not made to be with children, even their own, for the majority of their time. Some people are not made to slave away at a J-O-B for the majority of their time. We get into trouble when we try to do what doesn't feel good to us, so stay in the place that feels good to you.

Separation

Remember, "It takes a village . . ."? Well, our village has been dismantled by life's chaos and everyone is heading for the hills to figure it out on their own, causing us to feel disconnected from ourselves and from one another. We don't ask for help, and we judge those who do. So we attempt to do it all by ourselves, and we stress out.

Instead of managing this stress in healthy ways, we indulge in unhealthy behaviors, like skipping meals, overeating or eating unhealthy foods, numbing ourselves with drugs, lying awake in bed all night, or watching television. This has become the norm for far too many.

Hello! This is not serving us. We cannot do it all alone. We must reach out to one another for help. This separation must end.

Stress

Stress is a state of mental or emotional strain or tension resulting from a difficult or demanding circumstance.

According to Statistic Brain Research Institute and the American Institute of Stress in New York:
Seventy-seven percent (77%) of the population regularly experiences physical symptoms caused by stress.
Seventy-three percent (73%) of the population regularly experiences psychological symptoms caused by stress.
Fifty-six percent (56%) of the population lives with chronic stress.
Thirty-three percent (33%) feel they are living with extreme stress.

Are you among these numbers?

If we want to live longer, better, and happier, we must find a way to deal with stress because it is not going away. We must face it head-on and deal with what is causing the stress. However, we must also realize it is not all bad.

"Eustress" is the type of stress we feel when we're excited. This is the kind of stress we feel on a rollercoaster ride, when we're working on an important project, going on a first date, or waiting in anticipation for that first kiss. Acute stress is triggered by a surprise that requires a response. Eustress is acute stress, but it does not take a toll if we deal with it directly and return to a "stress-free" state.

However, "chronic stress" is the worrisome type. Chronic stress occurs when we repeatedly—90 days or more, according to experts—face stressors that take a toll and feel inescapable. A stressful job or an unhappy home life can bring on chronic stress and has devastating effects on our wellbeing. Our bodies are not designed to tolerate chronic levels of stress, so when we live this way, we become susceptible to dis-ease.

Today, we experience stress due to job pressure, money, health, relationships, poor nutrition, media overload, and sleep deprivation. Everyone is under stress, and we cannot avoid it. NOT dealing with stress is making us sick, our children sick, and the Material World sick. Our personal and professional lives are impacted negatively. We have difficulty managing our work and family responsibilities. We fight more with the people who are close to us. We alienate those we love, and we pay more for medical care. Chronic stress does devastating damage to our bodies.

Without much thought, we ask so much from our minds, bodies, and souls. We are walking, miracle beings and often neglect our most basic needs. Then, we demand more day-in and day-out to get through our incredibly busy days, where getting it all "done" is and has always been just a fantasy.

The sad thing is that we continue working as hard as we can until our bodies break down. We don't slow down until we don't have a choice.

Stress in and of itself is not the issue; the issue is how we deal with it. We must to let go of the things that stress us out, or we need to change the way we feel about them.

Unfortunately, most of us hand over control of our emotions to circumstances, situations, and other people. The truth is that we control the amount of stress we allow to invade our bodies and lives. If something in your life is stressing you and making you unhappy, change it. And as Maya Angelou says, "If you cannot change it, change the way you feel about it."

I know this isn't easy. But it is necessary. An absolute must. It is time to take responsibility for how you feel and understand that how you feel affects your wellbeing.

We Get Sick

Stress does devastating things to our body, mind, and soul.

Fatigue, headache, upset stomach, muscle tension, change in appetite, teeth grinding, change in sex drive, dizziness, irritability, anger, nervousness, lack of energy, and feeling as though you could cry have become the norm. Left untreated, these symptoms can cause greater issues.

Instead of dealing with our stressors, we opt for medication, pop a pill for this and that, thinking we cannot change our circumstances—but we can.

Our Children Get Sick

Our stress takes a toll on our families and children. Each month, almost one-third of children experience physical symptoms associated with stress.

According to the 2010 Stress in America Study, while 69% of Americans said their stress had no effect on their children, only 14% of children said their parents' stress had no effect on them.

What would your children say?

When children are stressed, they eat too much, sleep too much, and favor sedentary coping activities such as watching television. They frequently engage in bullying activities and don't do well in school.

Our World Gets Sick

When we are too exhausted and stressed to deal with daily life, everyone suffers. If we choose to feel good, then being our best selves isn't a chore.

If we think about why accidents happen, why people argue, why we aren't at peace, and why all these things we don't want in our lives happen, we can see they happen because we are not feeling good and not doing anything to feel better. We are not living from a place of love. We are living in the darkness of the chaos and fear that is perpetuated and reflected by what we choose to focus on in the Material World.

We say we want peace, but we look for and cause strife. We say we want to be healthy but don't nourish ourselves well. We say we want to be happy but make it the responsibility of the world to give us something to be happy about.

We must stop the madness and get a handle on the chaos of the Material World that impacts our capacity for health, wealth, and happiness, and that threatens our ability to thrive.

The Bottom Line

During The Illness, one of my biggest life challenges to date, I had the realization that I do not want to survive. Please hear me out, because I can't help but wonder: who just wants to survive?

Okay, yes. I am grateful I am here. But don't I owe it to myself, my family, society, the Material World, the Universe to do more than simply survive? That's like wanting only enough water to quench your thirst or only enough food for a meal. And of course, my favorite survivor thought…

I don't want much. I just want a little bit of money. Enough to buy a small house and pay off the bills so I can live out my days comfortably and in peace.

Really? That's going to give you comfort and peace?

Are you saying it because it sounds good or because you really mean it?

Your answer matters. If living in survival mode is all it takes to make you happy, fantastic. But if you have a strong desire that is calling from the inside to do more than survive, perk up, because you can achieve that too. What matters is that you have the courage to get out of your own way and go for what you want.

We don't all want the same things. Some people want more money. Some want simplicity. Others want more love. Still, others want it "all." There is nothing wrong with any of these choices. Only you can define what having it all and personal success mean to you.

Lighting the Way

Some say we are at a critical time in history when love and fear are colliding. If this is so, it's a good thing. We must live with passion, purpose, and play to receive the gift that life is.

When I was lost in the darkness of chaos, I thought I was alone. One of the most comforting things I learned was that I was not. I know that doesn't sound right, but it's the truth. Millions of people were—and are—going through something similar to what I experienced. As a result, more people are stepping out and stepping up to take center stage and share how they have transformed their Material World, how to live more deliberately, and how the change has impacted their lives for the better. For that, I am grateful.

Ariana Huffington, the author of *Thrive*, shared her story of literally passing out from exhaustion and waking up in a pool of blood, the unfortunate result of hitting her face on her desk on the way down and breaking her cheekbone. That was her wake-up call to creating a life worth living.

Brene Brown, the author of ***Gifts of Imperfection***, ***Daring Greatly***, and ***I Thought It Was Just Me, But It Isn't***, shared her story of feeling shame and judgment for being a working mom and how overwhelming the duties of motherhood were, along with pressures to perform.

Elizabeth Gilbert, the author of several books including ***Big Magic*** and ***Eat, Love, Pray***, shared her battle with fear, as she struggled to reconnect to a version of herself she could recognize.

There are so many stories of those who lost faith and found their way back, everyday people like you and me, figuring it out one day at a time, one step at a time.

Each story I hear leaves clues, much like parables, lessons to be learned and integrated, things we can do to make our lives more fulfilling and meaningful. I study these stories for clues, looking for patterns and the tale-tell signs of what makes someone feel bad or good, what inspires them, the limiting beliefs that hold them back, and the driving force to their accomplishments.

When I set out on my path to wellbeing, not even knowing then what I was doing, I did well over 1,000 hours of research. I wanted to know the best practices for creating a life worth living: what time to wake up, when to go to bed, how long to sleep, what to do in my spare time, how many hours to work, what to eat, when to eat, etc. In search of common threads to creating health, wealth, and happiness, I took notes on every aspect of every story I heard and read about healing and living well.

I remain obsessively committed to this passion—with many thanks to a peaceful movement fueled by those who are sick of surviving, living in the darkness of chaos, rising up to speak; with great thanks to people like Louise Hay and Oprah for shining a light on authors, doctors, experts, and everyday people like you and me, who have acquired information and wisdom to heal our souls so we may reclaim our birthright for total wellbeing.

We are seeing more and more role models, stepping out, living in alignment with who they are and what they want. They are very clear about their true desires and don't give into the chaos. These are the Spiritual Girls who know how to shine their light and calm the chaos of the Material World.

You give me hope because you are here, reading this book, open to different ways of thinking and doing, open to cleaning up decades of sloppy thinking that have caused dis-ease, dysfunction, and discomfort you no longer want to experience.

But we need more. Lots more.

The Real Deal

Most people ignore or are unaware of the actual consequences of our high-pressure, high-stress, and fast-paced lifestyles, and what they mean to our long-term quality of life. I've already been there and done that, so you can make the shift and stop the madness.

The Illness gave me the gift of clarity. Because my life was spared, my mission is to bring awareness to the devastating consequences faced when we neglect our wellbeing; to refocus our attention on the real value of living a life of quality; and to bring forth a way of life with passion, purpose, and play, while achieving true success without sacrificing your health, wealth, and happiness. The Material World is beautiful in its natural state, but that's not what we see. What we see are things that distract us from what matters most: our highest desires and wellbeing.

The people we interact with send us messages about what is important and how to live; they teach us what to believe. Our beliefs about how to live are further influenced by the 3,000+ messages we receive each day, telling us who we should be, what we should like, how we should act, where we should live, and how to be like the "happy" people. Along the way, we are never taught how to discern what we actually want. This bias bullies us into believing we are not enough as we are.

"Drink this shake and look great." "Wear these clothes, and you will be irresistible." "You just need this pill to sleep, that pill to have sex." Seriously? It's time to get back to the basics if we hope to create a life in which we achieve the success we desire without sacrificing our wellbeing.

Fear

When we experience challenge, struggle, or problems, we instinctively run. Or, we fall apart when things don't go our way. Then we ask, "Why me?" and take on the victim role. I'm sorry, but it's time for some tough love. See the fear. Feel the fear. Then move anyway. Don't allow fear to dictate your destiny. Everything worthwhile takes work and growth. It can be uncomfortable and is almost never easy. Sometimes, there's no way around this. And that's all right.

Overwhelm

Even with the internet and all the information available to us, there is still confusion about exactly how to create a life worth living, one in which you live passionately, purposefully, and playfully, without sacrificing your wellbeing.

Computers and other technology devices have taken over our lives like weeds in a flowerbed. They keep us from fully blooming, yet they are not the ones to blame. They were created to make our lives easier. Used unwisely, they wreak havoc in our everyday lives. It's time to look at technology and the related chaos in a new way, a way that serves what we sincerely desire.

It's Time

We must start doing things differently if we want different and better results. If we want to live more fully connected to our lives and feel amazing, then we must do things in alignment with that desire. If we want to savor those special moments, we must create time to reflect on them. If we want to enjoy the journey, we must create the time to celebrate the experiences that make us weak in the knees and tingle with warmth.

We cannot blame the Material World. We created it. We fuel it. We label it. We must reclaim our personal power and reclaim the responsibility for our health, wealth, and happiness if we hope to amplify our wellbeing.

A Spiritual Girl

Those who know, without question, what they want out of life are winners. When we are lost in our thoughts and dreams without action, we lose.

The inner workings of our health, wealth, and happiness are as complex as they are fulfilling. When we declare our desires and commit to them, incredible synchronicity happens. Some people call it luck. Whatever you call it, know you create it by living in alignment with the desires of your higher self.

A Spiritual Girl is someone who lives in complete alignment with her beliefs, desires, and values. Life does not happen to her. She does not live by default, taking what comes her way and never asking for more. She takes action each day, with commitment and dedication to what she wants to feel. She is open to life's experiences, without judgment or shame, so she can acquire wisdom to fulfill her destiny and live the way her soul intends, honoring her feelings and trusting her intuition to guide her to her desired destination.

The Others

Change does not happen through desire alone. Meditating, saying affirmations and lighting incense, setting intentions, and praying for what you want will not cause what you desire for yourself to come to fruition. You must take action and do the work.

"The Others" are individuals who act as blocks to achieving your desired reality. They are those people who judge you, fear for you, and caution you to be careful with your newfound courage. They are the people who tell you to be realistic and take off the rose-colored glasses.

Don't worry about The Others. You cannot control them or the way they think. You are better not to try. Live in the reflection of what you want and what you believe. Let nothing keep you from making your dreams your reality.

The Others, who live by default, will continue to struggle, unsure of what they are doing or where they belong, not showing up in life as their best and highest selves. They have no direction and give up the responsibility to fulfill their destiny or happiness. They continue to take life as it comes, allowing it to dictate their perceptions and affecting their ability to do more than survive from day-to-day. They merely survive in the Material World, feeling as if ease, luck, and success are never meant to be theirs.

The Awakening

Like so many of us, I was taught to hold in my feelings, never express emotion, and put on a happy face no matter how I felt. For decades, I practiced and mastered the art of appearance—an artform that enforces that sickness is synonymous with weakness, that the only way to be successful is by working hard to accumulate more and prove your worth, that feelings of fear, shame, resentment, anger, hurt, and overwhelm should be buried deep within. I became a master at masking them until I could cry them out, alone in the shower—because tears are never to be seen.

After working in the legal industry for twenty years, I acquired neurological Lyme disease that went undiagnosed for nearly four years. During that time, The Illness left me depleted, desperate, and eventually disabled.

My symptoms of pain, migraines, and insomnia became chronic and overwhelming. I became a statistic, another victim of my environment, a survivor in the strictest sense, but not a thriver. I gave up. I gave up my personal power and lost any illusion of control and responsibility over my wellbeing.

I was dying and disconnected. I stopped dreaming. I ceased having fun. I had lain in my bed for almost a year. I asked myself those big, end-of-life questions. Did I live passionately and on purpose? Did I matter to anyone other than myself? Did I make a difference in the world or in the lives of those who know me? Reflecting on what I did and did not do, I wondered if I had shown up more in love or in fear. Devastated and in dismay, I accepted my fate.

Except, it didn't happen. I didn't die. Instead, I was granted a new beginning. I transformed my mindset, created a plan to focus on what is important in my life, and learned to make myself a priority. I got myself out of that bed and back into a banging life. I have a lot to make up for, so I haven't stopped moving toward my desires since that day, one step at a time, with more intense focus than ever before.

I took that call from my doctor on February 11th, four months before my fortieth birthday, while I was in bed, as usual. He told me that my last blood tests, MRIs, ultrasounds, and bone marrow testing were all negative. They had revealed nothing of concern.

Feeling frustrated and alone, I took a deep breath and said, "Thank you," then hung up the phone.

At that moment, I dropped to my knees. I begged for answers. Why have I been unable to live a life of meaning for the last eighteen months? Why have I been confined to my bed for the better part of a year?

In a blacked-out fury, I cried. I yelled. I screamed. I threw and hit things. I scratched my face. I busted my knuckles and pulled out my hair with bloody hands. By the time I came back into my body, it was all done. I finally surrendered. I had no more fight left in me. All the illusions disappeared. I was ready. I gave up and for the first time, I realized why.

I had lost my vision, the vision of what I wanted my life to be. I had lived on automatic pilot, running myself ragged to keep up with the expectations of the Material World. Because I pushed to be all things to all people in my life—except myself—my wellbeing was compromised. It took years to return to some sense of normalcy.

My thoughts often return to the day I received that call from my doctor. I still cannot explain exactly why the shift in my thinking came at that time, but I am grateful it did. I was ready to rethink everything to create a life worth living, perhaps for the first time in my life.

I began to pour over studies, books, reports, white papers, interviews, and articles to grasp every golden nugget of wisdom available from specialists, doctors, psychiatrists, therapists, and expert authors on wellbeing.

Starting with nutrition, I made some drastic changes for my health. After three months of eating organically, detoxing, and juicing several times a day, I felt more alert, so much so that I started spending time in other areas of my house, not just my bedroom. I began doing things I had not done in nearly year, things like sitting on the sofa to watch a movie and reading a book by the pool.

My next step was to speak to my doctors about eliminating my medications. I felt toxic and wanted to get an accurate sense of where I was without the prescriptions. I was numbed and emotionally paralyzed. More than anything, I wanted to feel again.

While healing and addressing my physical symptoms, I considered what was happening to me mentally. Being unwell made me feel emotionally raw. Grief, depression, anxiety, resentment, shame, and fear in all its various forms had a firm grip on my state of mind. My research led me to why I was not well, and the way to heal myself became glaringly obvious. It was time to take a closer look at the way I lived.

As I integrated the information I was discovering into my lifestyle, along with the strategies, systems, and tools I was creating, I began to feel emotionally stronger and physically able to start participating in my life again.

As a result, I took a step back from my goals and what I thought, at the time, I wanted to achieve for myself. I considered first how I wanted to feel. Then, I thought about who and how I wanted to be. This helped me define what I had to do and how I had to live to feel the way I wanted to feel. No more sacrificing my long-term goals for short-term gains. I did not want to be influenced by my predefined roles or obligations as a woman, mom, employee, wife, sister, or daughter. I wanted to connect to the version of myself that I recognized: my best and highest potential as defined by ME.

I do things now that make me feel good and suited to my best and highest interests. Today, I attend and speak at conferences, events, and trainings hosted by the specialists, doctors, psychiatrists, therapists, and expert authors I have studied. Instead of creating goals based on what I want to acquire, I create goals based on how I want to feel. Everything I do in my life is based on amplifying my feelings of health, wealth, and happiness. For me, it is a whole new way to create a life worth living. It gives me meaning and fulfillment that I was always told could only be achieved in another life.

By evaluating my connection to everything around me, renegotiating my relationships, and trusting in the process of life again, I tuned into the person I knew in my gut I still had the potential to be. That's when the path to passion, purpose, and play revealed itself to me. Since that time several years ago, I have created and continue to create all the freedom, love, and laughter I once thought I didn't deserve. I wholeheartedly know you can do it too.

I forced myself to justify the *why* of everything in my life. If it felt good, I kept it. If it didn't feel good, I didn't. Cutthroat, yes, I know. But necessary. I was fighting for my life, and you are too, at least, your quality of life. From this place of clarity and deep understanding of what is necessary to achieve total wellbeing, I developed The Flight Plan, which I introduce in Chapter 2 and you will learn about in detail in Chapter 3. With it you will stay focused and on the path to creating a life worth living as defined by you, on your terms.

The Flight Plan is a life management system that helps you connect to your Inner Spirit so you can quiet the chaos of the Material World and achieve the success you desire without sacrificing your health, wealth, and happiness. I'm going to give you the steps to go from surviving to thriving so you can create a life worth living.

Chapter 2

Thrive by Design

"The unexamined life is not worth living."
~Socrates

If I had shared my story with you a few years ago, my point of view would not have been what it is now. My time-out, with many thanks to "The Illness," was a blessing, as challenges in our lives often are. From abuse to victimhood, hundreds of events and circumstances can make us feel as if life just happens and that we have no control over who or how we are, leaving us to ask whether these things occur for a reason. The reality is they are incidental and happen for us, not to us.

The range of my experiences has provided me with an abundance of knowledge and wisdom I appreciate. I don't feel sorry for myself or anyone else who has grown and evolved from their experiences. They empower us. It took me decades to realize I have a choice in how I experience my journey. I can look at my experiences through eyes of love and feel like a victor, or I can look through eyes of fear and feel like a victim.

There was a time about twelve years ago…

Just long ago enough for me to separate myself from it and recent enough to remember all the details.

I was an independent, working woman with a chip on my shoulder. Some consider the northwest side of Chicago, Illinois, where I grew up, the ghetto. But I have seen and experienced much worse. We were poor, but we were not destitute. I had a very light complexion compared to my family and those I lived around, so I had developed a thick skin.

I was miserable, and it was all my fault. I was getting less than five hours of sleep a night and working well over forty hours a week. I was as likely to ask you, "What the hell are you looking at?" as I was to wish you a good day. My mood was dependent on the traffic, the weather, and how much crap I had to get done that day.

From time to time, I would notice how much I had strayed from the path I dreamt of as a child. I wanted to be a marine biologist, living simply on a boat off some Caribbean island. But that was not to be my destiny. I worked in a law firm in Chicago, surviving and letting the day-to-day drama pile up and bury me alive with my dreams. A miserable attitude; hospital stays here and there; mistakes that led to consequences I was willing to pay for because I didn't know any better—these were my tolls for accepting survival as the default for living well in the Material World.

At the time, I didn't realize the signs that linked the path to my downfall. Looking back now, I see the clues and, as I share my story, I am sure you will recognize your signs too. I wish I could say everything started 12 years ago, but it didn't. My life was a cyclical breathing, living, and walking testament to what happens when you do not hold a vision for what you desire and perpetually follow the path of least resistance.

*In our pursuit of happiness, we must live from a good-feeling place,
if we want to live a truly successful life.*

I lived each day doing all the things I was told would make me
happy, yet I never felt good or fulfilled. I lived without much thought
about what I actually wanted to experience or feel. I didn't think
about myself from a loving perspective. I placed blame and didn't
take responsibility for creating a path that would allow me to live the
life my soul intended. I didn't feel worthy. I accepted what came my
way by default, even when it didn't feel good, as if I had no choices.
I made the best of what I got—or so I thought—just like everybody
else I knew.

I gave my power away when I was very young and didn't reclaim
it for decades. I never felt right in my skin. I gave until I had no
more to give. Then I gave up. My body, mind, and soul begged me
to STOP SURVIVING. It took decades, but I finally listened, and
this is my story of going from surviving to thriving.

My Story

Life was never what I would call easy. I was the daughter of teen
parents, growing up on the northwest side of Chicago in the early
1970s. My parents' marriage lasted only four years, but those four
years left an everlasting impression on me.

One of my first memories is watching a huge blow out between
my parents, then my mother's family rushing in to help her. It was
1974 and, shortly thereafter, my mom and I left for Puerto Rico
in hopes for a more peaceful life. I was only four, but I remember
feeling loved, safe, and cared for during the short time we were away.
Unfortunately, it didn't last. About a year later, we returned to the
states at the urging of my father who lured my mother back with a

promise of peace. The peace eventually came, but only after several more years of violence and drama.

My mom, Carmen, is a Puerto Rican woman from a family of twelve. My father, Michael, was an ethnic mix of English, Mexican, and German from a family of eight. Due to this racial combination, I witnessed and experienced racism from both ends of the spectrum. I never seemed white enough or brown enough to be accepted by either social group. My light skin, green eyes, and straight dark hair gave my mixed ethnicity away and made it difficult to fit in.

The Father – Michael

Michael grew up on the streets of the northwest side of Chicago. He is the second eldest in his family, born and raised in Chicago, Illinois, by Margaret and Paul, my grandparents. They are beautiful and compassionate people who worked hard to support their family.

I remember celebrating one of my birthdays at my grandparents' house on Fox Lake in McHenry, Illinois. Grandma bought me a cake with white frosting topped with Cookie Monster and Elmo sugar cookies. My father's six brothers and his sister were there. We took a boat out on the water that weekend, and I swam and played. It was a fun and beautiful day. That's my first birthday cake memory. I don't remember how old I was, all I remember was how loved I felt.

My grandparents are good people. I am blessed. I have a close relationship with my Grandmother, and until Grandpa's passing I had a close relationship with him too. We have had several conversations about their lives and challenges. I know they did the best they could do.

I don't recall Michael being around much when I was a child. This is one good memory. Today, I have a very complex and distant relationship with Michael so I don't have much to share about him.

The Mother – Carmen

Carmen is a dedicated big sister to her large family. She is third eldest of her three brothers and eight sisters. Born in Puerto Rico, she was brought to the States by her family for a better life. Maria and Roque, my Abuellos (grandparents in Spanish…to call them anything else would feel disrespectful) were magnificent people who worked hard to open a world of opportunity for their family.

I have endless memories with my Abuellos. My mom raised me near their home, and for most of my childhood, I would go to their house after school.

Carmen and Michael knew each other from the time she was nine, and they dated throughout high school. However, my conception was not to be celebrated. Devastated and ashamed to be pregnant at 18, Carmen ran away from home. Abuella found her and convinced her to come home. She did. Then she and Michael got married. Unfortunately, Carmen was kicked out of school for being pregnant, but she did earn her GED.

My parents divorced when I was four years old. By the time I was seven, Mother had married again, this time to a man who didn't like children, at least from what I could tell. She had another baby, my sister, Misty. Thank goodness, it was a short marriage. By the time I was nine, Mom was on her own again with another child to care for.

Mom did her best. We had more than most families in our neighborhood. We were poor, but many of my friends were really poor. We always had food, heat, and clothes; many of my friends did not. Mom was stressed out and, in time, developed her own way of disciplining me. She often bragged about how the monthly beatings kept me in line. I wish they would have worked, but they didn't. The beatings only made me angry, dismissive, and resentful of anyone who tried to exercise authority over me.

One time, when I was about six, I was going downtown with my aunt and my cousins to see the big Christmas tree and window displays at Marshall Fields and Carson Pirie Scott. On the way to the train, I fell in the snow. My aunt sent me back home because my coat was covered in mud. When I returned to the house in tears, my mother yelled and hit me for getting dirty. It got so bad that one of my other aunts threw herself on top of me and begged my mother to stop.

I wish I could say this was my only or worst story, but it isn't. There were lots of incidents that I'll spare myself recalling and you the details.

More would come my way as I was molested by a man my mother trusted, and knew me since the day I was born. It started slowly, when I was ten, and increased in severity and frequency from there. When I was in sixth grade, I went to his place for a visit, and he slept with me that night. By morning, I had experienced another hurt that weighed me down for decades to come.

Again, I wish I could tell you this was the only instance, but it wasn't. I wish I could say he was the only man to betray my trust, but he wasn't. Between the beatings and sexual abuse, there wasn't much I would not do to escape my life.

But I didn't say anything. I didn't think anyone would care, so I didn't reach out. I just looked for a way out. Before my teen years, I took off for days at a time. I became consensually sexually active when I was thirteen, so it should not have surprised me when I got pregnant at fifteen. But, of course, it was. I was a sophomore in high school and my boyfriend, seventeen, was a dropout.

I started my junior year of high school with a newborn baby, Miggie, and a new attitude. This was my wake-up call to completely change my ways and my life. I was going to do for this baby what I felt my parents did not do for me.

Like my mother, I was a teen mom. But I wanted my daughter's story to be different. I was going to support her emotionally. I was going to let her know she is always loved unconditionally. I was going to give her all the things I felt were missing in my life.

I worked nights and weekends to make ends meet while I went to school full-time. Fred, her father, did his part too. Out of necessity, Fred moved into my mother's house just before Miggie was born. Things were complicated, to say the least. We did our best.

I have to admit, while I'm happy I made it, I would never want to relive this time in my life. Things felt impossible then. I had little hope for happiness. I graduated from high school and went to college full-time while continuing to work part-time. I didn't have much more to give. While everything on the outside seemed fine, by the time I was twenty, I was miserable but still doing what had to be done.

A rare opportunity appeared: a graduate-level, certified paralegal training program that was being opened to college students. To get in, students needed a good grade-point average, at least a year's worth of college credits, and an attorney sponsor. Applicants also had to survive a panel interview. I did it. I made it in. It took me nine months of going to school and working six days a week, but I finished. I graduated from the paralegal program that would allow me to support my daughter without all the struggles I'd been experiencing. Immediately after graduating, I got a new job and doubled my income.

All I ever wanted for our family was to live in a good, safe neighborhood; to have a good car that would get us from point A to point B without any problems; to give my daughter a great education; and to live in a nice home. By the age of twenty-three, I did all that, along with her father and my soon-to-be husband.

Fred, my daughter's father, and I married in 1993. In 1996, we had twins, Roque and Reyna, children we planned and had together. As you can imagine, motherhood was quite a different experience this go-round.

Once again, I had something new to strive for. I wanted to do better for my family. Fred soon had a new career as a tattoo artist, and I continued working as a commercial real estate paralegal.

By the time the twins were seven, I was nervous about living in Chicago. My mother still lived in the same neighborhood I grew up in. Although it's a beautiful city, I knew I could not raise a son in the streets where I was raised. I never wanted him to face the kind of violence I had. So, we left.

By far, this is one of the hardest things I have done. I left my whole family behind: my parents, sister, uncles, aunts, and cousins. Despite our difficult history, in my adult years we had lots of good times and we grew into such a close family. I loved the times we spent together, but I had to go.

In 2004, we moved to Orlando, Florida. Migdalia, my eldest, almost eighteen at the time, came with us. The twins, Roque and Reyna, were eight.

That Was Then

If I had known then what I know now, I would not have left my hometown. That's the truth. I realized no matter how often I returned, the distance grew between my family and me. I was so ignorant. I never thought this would happen. The cards and invitations stopped coming within a couple of years. Then when I got sick and had to stop visiting, communication was nearly cut off. To this day, many of those relationships have not been mended. I look back on those times in Chicago fondly and am so grateful for those experiences. That's the extent of what I carry in my body, mind, and soul from this period in my life.

After the move to Florida, I started to feel the pressure to make a new life for my family. I worked hard to deliver what everyone needed. There was a time, about one year after the move, when I considered going back home to Chicago. But the twins loved Florida, and Miggie was in school and making new friends.

I worked a lot of hours, often leaving the home and family care to Fred as I worked late into the evening. As usual, I felt compelled to prove my worth. I worked well over forty hours a week. On weekends, I entertained and took the kids out for a good time. Orlando provided us with endless options. The guilt I felt over not being enough fueled my exhausting schedule as I tried to live up to the enormous expectations I had created for myself.

In 2008, after I had struggled with chronic pain and fatigue for two years, the pain pills had taken their toll on my body. I had to have my colon removed. I should have recovered in eight weeks, but it took me four years.

By 2009, I was no longer driving or working. The doctors experimented with my medications to help me find the right combination simply to get me through the day. With an eventual cocktail of eleven medications, we were unsuccessful.

During this time, I went to therapy. I needed someone to talk to about all the secrets I had stored as nested treasure chests, hidden deep in my belly. That's how I imagined the memories haunting me. I could no longer keep these memories locked away. Being exhausted and in pain didn't leave me with the strength required to keep those treasure boxes locked and buried.

Worn down and burnt out, all my secrets were flooding out of me. I could no longer hold the pain and emotion that went along with all the anger, resentment, and shame I felt for decades.

I was *so* angry. I was angry with my parents. I was angry with my extended family. I was angry with friends. I was angry with my husband. But most of all, I was angry with myself. I had no love, and I started to think my husband and children would be better off without me. I would never say I was suicidal, but there were nights when I prayed that I wouldn't wake up.

I was depleted, depressed, and disabled. I felt like no one cared, like my life had no meaning, and that everyone had forgotten about me. I thought I was dying. I gave up my vision of what life could be. I wasn't sure I wanted to try. I didn't see the worth in my life anymore, and wondered why everything was so hard.

The Gift

The Illness gave me the ability to dream, to dream a bigger dream, a new vision of what health, wealth, and happiness—my wellbeing— could mean to and for me. That was my gift. No longer would I wait for the approval I had craved ever since I had disappointed myself by getting pregnant at fifteen. I was finally free of the weight of that guilt and ready to discover what I wanted to leave as *my* legacy.

Why had I been content to simply survive?
Why didn't I dream a bigger dream for myself, for my life?
Why didn't I want to be like Madonna and roll on stage, singing "Like a Virgin"?
Why didn't I want to be like Marianne Williamson and speak about returning to love?
Why didn't I want to be a world-class attorney and close the biggest real estate deals in the country?

I have always been a high achiever. Most teen moms from inner city Chicago don't make it to where I was when The Illness took over. By the age of thirty-seven, I had accomplished all my goals. I was successful by the definition of success I had established for myself.

Looking back now, I realize I was expecting to stay there, retire, and then finish my days. I couldn't think of the future because I had no more dreams. There was nothing else for me. I was coasting along, living the "dream," the biggest one I had ever had. The problem is that it didn't feel like a dream; it felt more like a nightmare. I felt like a caged animal looking to escape and be free.

To reclaim my sense of freedom and wellbeing, I went on a journey like none other in my life. I made myself well, and I created a new vision for my life, new dreams to dream, new ideas to explore, new goals to achieve.

This is Now

I started my journey by being honest about where I was. Then I was ready to get informed.

First, I researched each of my symptoms and what I could do to improve them. I wanted off the medications. I read books, reports, and white papers. I spoke to doctors and fellow patients. I searched and read everything I could on the web, looking for solutions.

At some point, my research moved from my pain to my life and led me to ask the bigger questions. Finally, the biggest question of all came to me.

How can I create a life worth living?

How can I create a life where I would never be abused, judged, or shamed? A life where I have the courage to live from my heart and follow my gut? A life where I do what I enjoy for work and play? A life where every day is filled with passion, purpose, and play?

Not a life someone else told me to live.

I wanted the recipe for creating a life that was completely fulfilling and meaningful, based on what I wanted to be and feel. I was tired of The Others dictating to me what I needed. More importantly, I was ready to take responsibility for my health, wealth, and happiness.

By reading the stories of how others overcame their obstacles and challenges, I learned so much. I created best practices, boundaries, and strategies from their stories. My research taught me about using meditation for pain, something that worked well for me and was a great alternative to prescription pills. I learned to sit for up to two hours at a time in meditation for my pain, when necessary. As I continued my research, I felt an intuitive call to strengthen my spirituality.

I left my religion when I was pregnant with the twins. It was a difficult pregnancy. I was on bed rest from the time I was four months pregnant until I gave birth. I always felt ashamed and judged for who I was and how I lived. However, I prayed often and wanted to find a way to commune with a higher power. This is what led me to a little book I love and carry with me everywhere: ***You Can Heal Your Life***, by Louise Hay.

What stood out to me in ***You Can Heal Your Life*** is the index of symptoms and affirmations. For each symptom, Hay provides a description of why you may be experiencing it, with an affirmation to help heal your physical response to your emotional experiences. When I said the affirmations for each of my symptoms, I experienced relief.

This led me to start focusing on what I feel as a way to confirm I am on the right path. When I feel good, I know I'm in the right place; when I don't, I'm not. Usually, we measure our accrued power and money to know whether we are doing the right thing or living the right way. We don't use feeling and meaning. It struck me how simple this is and how much we love to complicate things.

The reality is the Material World is not to blame for the chaos. Our lack of clarity distracts us from the simplicity that life truly is and that isn't the Material World's fault. It's ours. So, it is time to get clear about who you want to be, what you want to do, and how you want to feel.

We complicate things by not using the Material World to our benefit. We bend and mold our lives to suit it rather than the other way around. We don't utilize the many options of the Material World in a way that feels good to us. We continually throw away our happiness by releasing the responsibility for it. We live like The Others, like the way they tell us to even though they are no closer to true success or happiness.

Taking inventory of where I was, why I was there, and how I felt about it was brutal. When you assume responsibility for your life, you have to ask, "*What has been my part in this?*" It is not always easy to face the facts, but it is necessary for real transcendence. I did my best not to place blame or judgment on myself or anyone else. I looked at the various life situations I didn't feel good about and imagined what I could have done differently, rather than what I might have done wrong. This is crucial to preventing blame and guilt. This allowed me to move forward and drop decades of baggage filled with anger, pain, and resentment.

We are taught that we cannot have it all. Yet, in the hope that we can, we grasp at anything we believe will lift us up. I am going to show you how to focus on the right opportunities, because you can have it all, on your terms, and as I've discovered, without sacrificing your wellbeing.

We learn we cannot achieve balance, but we kill ourselves trying. I am going to show you how to achieve balance because it does exist. Although it may not look the same for everyone, it is achievable. I'm going to show you how to define your purpose so you can create the balance you crave.

We learn we're crazy for trying something new, but we try and try anyway because there's a sense deep inside of us that knows trying new things is how we grow. I am going to show you how to prove yourself sane and create opportunities for the things you want to experience.

I used what I learned from my research to create The Flight Plan, which I share with you so you can create a life YOU love. I had to change up my original system for achievement because my highly effective and efficient process for getting the work done was missing some critical components. It was missing connection, compassion, and celebration. I never took time out for a pat on the back. I was too busy moving on to the next thing. I didn't make my connections to myself or my family a priority; I didn't have time for friendships. I had no compassion. I'd been through so much that I couldn't see or honor anyone else's struggle.

I cultivated a Thriving Mindset through Living with Passion. I discovered my priorities by Living with Purpose. This allowed me to align my desires and productivity by Living with Play. I was able to hush those not-so-quiet voices, insisting that I had all I deserved, that I needed to be satisfied with what life gave me, and that I should keep living by default. Gone are the feelings of sadness, loneliness, abandonment, shame, and fear. I have found love, unconditional and all-consuming. It's a beautiful thing to live in the magic and mystery of synchronicity, which is the result of calming the chaos.

I share this with you to show you how I saw the signs but ignored them. Losing my career and my sense of self was unnecessary. I see that now with a clarity I did not have before. I don't want anyone to visit the dark places I went in my mind when I was not well.

Now it's your turn to begin the journey. Wherever you are today on your journey to create a life worth living, it's time to go for the next level of happiness, health, and wealth that exists for you. Because I promise you, another level exists. You will reflect on how you got where you are only so you know where you need to go to get what you want. I will meet you wherever you are and guide you through The Flight Plan so you can define and forge your path.

I have worked with attorneys, doctors, financiers, business and life coaches, consultants, entrepreneurs, stay-at-home moms, and working women from all walks of life. As I taught them The Flight Plan, as I'm going to teach you, they have cleared the barriers that prevented them from achieving the success they desire in their careers and personal lives. They released limiting beliefs that held them back and created new empowering beliefs that propelled them to new levels of business and personal success. I have been honored and privileged to work with each of them and witness them take flight and soar.

Listen Up

Scattered throughout this book, you'll find sections marked "Moving Forward." These are stories from some of my clients (whose names have been changed to respect their privacy) who experienced incredible breakthroughs while taking their lives from surviving to thriving with The Flight Plan.

I have hundreds of "Moving Forward" stories, from people who thought they were stuck in lives with no control over their happiness. But because they were willing to think a different way, do different things, and commit to creating a life they love, they reclaimed their personal power and transformed the way they experience their world.

And make no mistake. This is about you creating the life experience YOU want for yourself.

So now, I ask you:

Do you listen when your body, mind, and soul speak to you?

Really. Do you?

This is just between you and you, so be real. Do you listen when your head hurts, when you can't catch your breath, when your heart palpitates, when your stomach flips, or when you can't sleep? Do you listen?

Moving Forward – Jennifer

Jennifer is a mompreneur, a mom and successful entrepreneur. On the outside, life seemed to be going well for Jennifer but she didn't feel good about it. She is blessed with a beautiful family and an amazing husband. She has wanted for nothing, yet, a part of her was preventing her from truly enjoying it. She often felt depressed and didn't know why. Honestly, I was surprised the day she reached out to me, two years ago.

When Jennifer created her Flight Plan, she realized she had no idea what she loved. She had lost her sense of preference and completely disconnected from the things that excited her. Her entire life was wrapped around making her home a happy place for her children and husband, but she did nothing to make it a happy place for herself. She left no spare moments and didn't take the time to enjoy the success she achieved.

Creating her Flight Plan empowered Jennifer to discover things that she loved again. She opened up to trying new hobbies and foods. She created a meditation space in her home and started painting and creating designs for her t-shirt business. Three months ago, Jennifer sold her little t-shirt business for $1.19 million. She now consults with the buyer on a part-time basis and provides designs on commission.

The Busyness

Love and honor yourself by taking a good and deep look at how you feel about what is going on around you. We must stop busying ourselves with what others tell us is important. It's time to do what feels important, from a wellbeing perspective, to create a life worth living. By digging into what we want to achieve and how we want to feel in our lives, we are better able to manage our power, priorities, and productivity. Living more intuitively allows you to create a life worth living without sacrificing your wellbeing. This is not about you conforming to what I feel good about. It is about discovering what makes you feel good.

I am very ambitious, passionate, organized, efficient, and productive. My life is what I call full, not busy. Yes, there are days when I don't get a chance to sit for more than a few minutes at a time; for me, that's the way it's supposed to be. I have a very clear purpose; I don't want to sit around waiting to see what happens. I want to do my part and make big things happen.

But that's not everyone. We all have different ebbs and flows, and through The Flight Plan, we'll define what having it all is and what living with passion, purpose, and play means to YOU. Allowing your feelings to guide you enables you to dismiss dis-ease and to steer your actions to accomplish your deepest desires so you can transform the way you experience your world.

Too often things like guilt, unforgiveness, and lack of presence keep us from fulfilling our hearts' true desires. And, in my opinion, fulfilling your heart's desire is your job here. At some point, each of us seeks to define our purpose to create depth, fulfillment, and meaning in our life.

Life is amazing, joyous, exciting, and so much more than I could ever articulate in this book. We forget this as we live in the blinding chaos and noise of the Material World. Everything that we experience, from the birds that fly above us to the trees that line our streets, is miraculous. This includes you; it includes everyone and everything. Owning your specialness has nothing to do with superiority. It has everything to do with equity so each and every one of us can rise to serve the best and highest version of ourselves.

What we are talking about is your wellbeing and creating a lifestyle that supports your wellbeing, as measured by the quality of your connections, health and wellness, achievement, organization, and spirituality, so that you can knowingly take action that will lead you, step-by-step, to achieving what you want.

To overcome the challenges and resistance around creating a life I love and that's worth living, I created what I call "Spiritual Prescriptions." I teach these Spiritual Prescriptions to my clients and share them worldwide when I speak as the Wellbeing Messenger.

I was a very sickly person until 2014, much of which stemmed from my busyness. Due to my diagnoses of neurological Lyme disease and epilepsy, I experienced seizures under physiological distress. I got colds that lasted months. I would lose my voice for weeks at a time, for seemingly no reason. I had asthma attacks several times a year. I was admitted to the hospital for at least one week every year for various unknown reasons. This was my life.

I remember seeing posts on social media saying, "Let Go," "Forgiveness is the Gift You Give Yourself," or "Just Be Happy." It sounded like a load of crap. I just didn't get it and couldn't get there. Or my favorite, when people tell you, "You just need to get in a good-feeling state." Seriously? If I could, I would.

The Flight Plan has helped me prioritize my wellbeing, and for the last two-and-a-half years, I have been much healthier. I have not had a seizure or even a single cold, which is a miracle considering I have flown over thirty times in the last couple of years alone.

When I am not feeling well or am what I call low vibe, I look to my Spiritual Prescriptions to address the issue, align myself, and keep moving forward. My Flight Plan keeps me from getting swallowed by the devouring chaos created by lack of clarity and by our Material

World, with its multimedia, apps, devices—the things that are supposed to make life feel easier.

I credit The Flight Plan for this health, wealth, and happiness in my life. The better I do at maintaining my wellbeing, the better I do at keeping my internal, aligned state clear of any resistance and emotional blocks. I live each day in alignment with what I desire. I know what I want, and I know where I am going. I accept full credit and responsibility for how I show up in the Material World. My actions, not my circumstances or experiences, define my legacy.

Surprises

Unexpected things happen in our lives. When they do, we must put The Flight Plan to work. Doing this work and having a Thriving Mindset doesn't mean I am immune to life's struggles. It means I honor them. I implore you to do the same.

Take 2013 to 2014 for instance. I lost seven people in my life, including one of my best friends, my Abuella, two cousins, and an aunt. These were people I thought of or interacted with daily. Before The Flight Plan, I would have been lost in the darkness of despair. I was surprised to find myself well, being of service to those who were struggling. I felt honored to be in that state of wellbeing and complete balance so I could serve my family and friends.

I was able to take swift action, have difficult discussions with clear communication, and feel well at the same time. I never sacrificed my ethics or integrity. These were sorrowful, heavy days for me, but my internal state of alignment was constant. When I felt drained, I took a break, listened to music and journaled, meditated, or prayed. All things I wouldn't have thought to do before The Flight Plan. I returned fully restored and ready for what was next.

Understand we cannot control what comes into our lives, but we can control how we respond to them. Everything I have learned about living well and balanced has made life exciting again. I no longer submit to the everyday drama that used to drain my batteries and bring chaos to my front door.

Honor yourself in a way that speaks to your soul.

Prepare to Create a Life Worth Living

What we are talking about here is creating a lifestyle that incorporates all the essentials for a well-lived life. To help you do that, I share in this book my unique lifestyle management system called The Flight Plan.

I created the Flight Plan as a practical way to live in alignment while creating a life worth living. It is one in which you are empowered to reclaim your time, calm the chaos, and transform the way you experience the Material World. It is one in which you can live with passion, purpose, and play. It is one in which you can achieve success without sacrificing your health, wealth, and happiness—not so you can *do* more, so you can *enjoy* more.

Section 2

WHERE DO YOU WANT TO GO?

Once you understand where you are, you have a starting point, a way to acknowledge growth and preference. Once you know what you don't want, learning what you do want is easier.

What does success look like in your life?

In the next three chapters, you will transform the way you experience your world, calm the chaos, and reclaim your precious time.

In Chapter 4, you will adopt a Thriving Mindset, because what you think is as important as what you do.

In Chapter 5, you will calm the chaos that distracts you from what matters to you most so you succeed on your terms and with health, wealth, and happiness.

In Chapter 6, you will reclaim your time and start investing it in happitunities that make the difference between surviving and thriving.

Chapter 3

The Flight Plan

"No one saves us but ourselves. No one can and no one may. We ourselves must walk the path." ~Buddha

Do you see the sadness in the fact that the skills to create a life worth living are never taught to us?

We learn that success is all about luck, the circumstances we are born into, and the balance in our bank accounts. We are stuck believing that we are where we belong and that anyone who breaks out is just fortunate by chance.

Reading, writing, and arithmetic will always be necessary elements of a comprehensive education. But, on their own, they do not equip you with the ability to lead a joyous and well-balanced life. In the traditional education system, there are no personal development classes for finding what you love to do, for healing, forgiveness, or for teaching us to love more and fear less. We are left to figure it out on our own. Most of us think a life worth living comes from working hard and playing harder. And for you, that may feel right, but there is more to creating a life worth living filled with depth and meaning.

People like to say, "Live every day like it's your last," but what does that get you? Living recklessly? Exhausted and fed up with all that hasn't worked out for you? That promotion you never got? That lover who left you instead of working it out? The weight you could never get rid of once and for all? Making decisions only thinking about now without consideration for tomorrow?

I say, "Live every day as if it's your *first*," engaging the same curiosity you originally carried into this world and filling your days with energy, enthusiasm, and excitement for what is to come. Look forward to getting the job of your dreams; to finding that lover who understands you and doesn't give up on you; to feeling so secure that you release extra weight and live healthily; to making decisions with your end in mind, knowing what you want to experience and feel along your journey.

I have words to remind myself of how I want to show up and to keep me tuned into the legacy I want to leave. I want to be loving, passionate, and present. I want people to say I am inspiring, caring, and engaged. Each day, I gauge how I am doing at living up to my words by checking my routines, my productivity, and my embodiment of those words.

What are your words?
How do you want to be described?
How will you check to make sure you are living in alignment?

The good news is that you hold all the power. Awareness empowers you to identify the time-suckers and energy-wasters, who consume your precious inner resources, and frees you to flex your mental, physical, and emotional wellness muscles, allowing you to clear the way for the important things—you know, those things that embody your joy and give your life incredible depth and meaning.

Living from this place, as if it's my first day, keeping who and how I want to be in mind, reminds me to respect my deepest, most loving desires. This allows me to honor the person I am and not that crazed woman who used to come out during trying times, lashing out and hurting people with her actions, intentions, and words.

One of the reasons I share my story with you is so you can see how changing my mindset saved my life. Believe me when I tell you that I went from feeling life's energy escaping my body to, the next day, feeling life's energy enter. The sensations were beyond description. I felt reborn, as if the hard shell that prevented anything good from coming in had cracked open.

I never looked back. I allowed the feeling to carry me. I decided to take another shot at life. No more surviving. I was tired of being sick and tired. I was going to live full out and be a loving, passionate, and present person. I reconciled with the fact that as long as there is air in my lungs and a heart beating in my chest, I am alive, and I will behave like it.

It is time to calm the chaos, my friend. As a society, we are exhausted, and any motivation to maximize productivity is generated by fear. We must look at productivity in a whole new way if we want to engage in a way of life that can be sustained long-term.

Life can get lonely and make us feel like our existence is just that: existence, survival, nothing special. We live and die. I believe there is much more than that. But even if you accept this philosophy, why wouldn't you want to make this the best damn life?

We are all special. Think of the miracle it took to bring you into being. Two people at exactly the right time had to come together to create the miracle that is you. That's pretty special, isn't it?

I know it doesn't always feel that way, but a sure way to feel good more often is to tune in to the miraculous being that is you. I need you to feel worthy of creating a life worth living. That is what each of us is promised when we are created and born into this world: the opportunity to create a life worth living. Nothing more, nothing less. If we continue dancing in the darkness of chaos in the Material World, living by default, allowing The Others to define our path, operating out of tune with our passion or purpose, we will not notice when we stray from our chosen path; life will feel hard, and we will question if it's worth the effort we put into it.

The Flight Plan is a way of living, a process you practice each and every day that keeps you aligned with your chosen path. Together, the three critical components of The Flight Plan create total wellbeing, allowing you to live more effortlessly with passion, purpose, and play to achieve the success you desire without sacrificing your health, wealth, and happiness.

Components of the Flight Plan

There are three critical components of the Flight Plan: Passion, Purpose, and Play. The upcoming sections explore how to live with Passion, Purpose, and Play, providing a clear understanding of how you infuse your Flight Plan with each component so you can achieve success without sacrificing your wellbeing.

Passion | Too many of us are disconnected from what we want and from the parts that make up our magnificence. We must foster the kind of passion that pulls us through to our next big adventure when we know, without question, how we want to experience life.

When I talk about Living with Passion, I am speaking of living in a way that honors the miraculousness of your existence and your highest desired potential. Too often, we close the passionate parts of ourselves. We feel selfish and indulgent when we focus on our desires, but this is not a self-centered or extravagant effort. Living with Passion is highly necessary if we want to live the best life we can. We all want that. We may not be able to articulate it, but it's what we all deeply desire: to live passionately.

We do this by Adopting a Thriving Mindset. Living with Passion prevents us from being a martyr for our success. Today, many of us live in fear and give in to fearful beliefs and thought patterns. The thoughts that enter our minds are based on our beliefs. Our actions are based on our thoughts. Hence, our lives are a direct reflection of the quality of those beliefs. To transform the way we experience the Material World, we must think differently.

Purpose | Most of us have no plan other than to show up and do our time each day. Wasting it, killing it, doing anything we can do with time other than investing it to bring more joy and ease into our lives. We must live with focus on what matters most. We must ignore the distractions that keep us from realizing our dreams and our highest desired potential. We must develop the kind of purpose that propels us out of bed each day.

In the Material World, it's easy to get lost in the chaos. We are overexposed to advertising, mass media, and social media. We receive thousands of messages each day, telling us who to be, what to wear, what to want, and how to live. Everyone is filled with advice about what you need, but they don't talk about HOW to live joyously. They don't talk about connection, health, achievement, organization, or spirituality in a way that creates depth and meaning in our lives.

Living with Purpose means doing the things that matter to you, the things that impact your desire for fulfillment and meaning. When calming the chaos with connection, health and wellness, achievement, organization, and spirituality, you design a life that feels good to YOU. This is your ultimate purpose.

Play | We must stop doing things we don't enjoy because of what they get us. Living this way has taken us down a path that doesn't feel good or meaningful. Our power to generate happiness has been handed over to the cashier, the traffic, the technology, the chaos. Thus, we must create the kind of play that is fun while getting the work done. Work is not a bad word; work is an effort directed to produce or accomplish something good. By redefining our work, we can turn it into play and enjoy more of the journey.

Life is supposed to be fun, and we are meant to play every day. In all the chaos and confusion of the Material World, we forget this. Every one of us is busy, but what are we actually achieving in this constant state of busyness? Are we doing the things that are important to us or doing things that are important to others? We have responsibilities we must take care of; however, we have only one life, so we must also enjoy how we invest our time.

The Material World makes it nearly impossible to focus on what really matters. Each of these Elements of Total Wellbeing calms the chaos that is unleashed upon us each day. By staying centered in your purpose, you learn to utilize technology and information to serve you, not sabotage you.

Moving Forward – Gisele

Gisele grew up with wealth and was told her entire life she could have anything she wanted. During her teen years and early 20s, her life felt complete with partying, shopping, and traveling. But in her mid-20s, she found herself in an emotional crisis and searched for something, anything that would make her feel happy, including drugs.

Gisele saw me speak at a conference and called me three days later. She asked if I could help her find a way to be happy with her life. We met the next day. During our first session, I asked her about what she wanted for herself. After a long thoughtful pause, she said, "I don't know."

She explained she had been doing what others told her brought them happiness, trying to replicate it in her own life, but nothing had worked for her. I immediately knew Gisele needed to define what a fulfilling and meaningful life felt and looked like for her without outside opinions and fear of judgment.

Gisele created her Flight Plan as I guided her to define what happiness in her life could look and feel like. We did a lot of work to discover her true desires and preferences. Within three months, Gisele created the feeling she had been searching for her entire life. Once she defined and allowed herself to discover and honor what made her feel the way she wanted to feel, happiness became a constant in her life.

We have been working together for two years. Gisele still uses her Flight Plan and is discovering things she never thought she would be open to. She also just had her first baby.

Health, Wealth, and Happiness

Before we move on, let's go over what creating a life worth living, filled with health, wealth, and happiness, means so that we are operating from a common place.

Health speaks to your state and level of care for your mental and physical wellness. This involves how you think, how you respond to life, and how you fuel your body.

Wealth speaks to the quality of your life experiences and connections. This has nothing to do with the accumulation of material things. Admittedly, allowing material things we find comfort in brings ease and good feelings, but it does not mean they are the end-all and be-all in achieving true wealth.

Happiness speaks to the level of joyous energy, engagement, and enthusiasm you exude through your state of being, your essence.

Happiness is your birthright and requires only your commitment. You only need to decide emphatically that you want to live well and will commit to doing what it takes.

We will be looking at what is lacking in your life, by your terms. Know you don't have to choose between having more connections, health and wellness, achievement, organization and spirituality. It is safe to have and want it all.

Release the judgment of those who decide not to live like you. We are all unique in our expression of life. That's what makes us beautiful, walking miracles.

When we live in a state of deliberate creation, things start to happen. Momentum starts building, taking us closer to the things that we want. We become "lucky" (and no, it is not random). Opportunities come to us. People are nicer. We get more things for free and with ease. It's pretty cool. Good things happen with little or no extra effort. It still shocks me and makes me laugh when I witness it. Being present to the miracles of life brings the most incredible faithfulness in the process of life.

Through the processes and elements that make up The Flight Plan, you will be empowered to create connection, health and wellness, achievement, organization, and spirituality to achieve and maintain total wellbeing and calm the chaos. Reclaim your personal power so you can define and create your legacy by design rather than by default. Proclaim and commit to your priorities based on the destiny you desire. Protect your productivity so you create the time to do what you want, when you want. Bring yourself back whenever you get lost in the dark chaos of the Material World so you don't spend any more of your precious time on the busyness and can, instead, invest it in creating a life worth living.

One of the most challenging things for me to do is find the right words to adequately articulate how living this way makes us incredibly joyous. Quite frankly, there aren't enough superlatives available. But here are some of the things that happen: You make better decisions. You stop noticing the small stuff and recognize their insignificance. You show up to be of service from a giving and loving place, not from obligation or through guilt. You feel happy and get more to be happy about.

You may think I'm getting a bit carried away here, but take it from this Spiritual Girl, it's freakin' AMAZING, and you will experience this. So, let's get into how you create this synchronicity in your life so you can soar too.

Bringing the Elements Together

The Flight Plan empowers you to define your purpose and to create goals for what they make of you, not what they get for you. By letting your purpose drive your actions, you build the momentum you need to achieve the success you desire without making sacrifices that compromise your wellbeing.

The Flight Plan empowers you to live from your soul. It requires that you want to be propelled out of bed each day, filled with excitement and enthusiasm. It requires that you let your passion fuel your dreams and loves in life. Living with Passion empowers you to change the lens through which you view what you experience, shifting it from a fearful to a loving perspective.

The Flight Plan empowers you to enjoy how you invest your time, and through The Keys I share with you, you will reclaim hours of your day and days of your life by taking action you enjoy on what matters most. The Keys will keep you moving forward so you never feel stuck again.

The Flight Plan allows you to focus on what matters, when it matters. It keeps you moving with inspired action to create a life worth living as defined consciously by you.

Preparation

You will be guided and supported through each component of The Flight Plan. Don't get hung up on the process. All you have to do is be present by living in the moment, suspending thoughts about your past and your future, and do the work. Exercises, which I call Spiritual Prescriptions, will help you identify and overcome challenges that are holding you back. Each prescription includes everything you need to calm the chaos so you can once again connect to the amazing love that exists within in you and the Material World.

Creating a life worth living is simple, but it isn't easy. I don't want to pretend it is. Before we get started with the chaos detox and exercise your thriving muscles, we must prepare for the journey. Here are a few things you need to know as you begin.

Accept Where You Are

Life is filled with peaks and valleys. We must learn to be okay with where we are. Each life experience teaches us a lesson we are here to learn. The challenges we face are opportunities to grow. Without them, life would be boring. You must have faith that you are experiencing what you need to experience to grow as a person. For some, it is a hard pill to swallow. I know. However, when you do, it's a lot easier to accept your experiences for what they are: growth opportunities.

As you embrace this new way of living, new people will come into your life. Others will leave. Know this is a natural process. Many people will not understand what you are doing for yourself or why. They will take personally your desire to transform your life.

Expect your friends and family to lack understanding about what you are doing. Likely, they are used to pretending everything is fine when it's not, and they probably give in to weak thoughts like The Others and participate in bad behaviors like gossiping and numbing. Expect them to bring you bad or upsetting news, telling you, "You can't always be happy." They may make assumptions about how you feel and react in haste by telling you, "You can't change who you are."

Know they are doing their best to support you and just don't get it—yet. As you make your shifts by adopting a Thriving Mindset and embodying the positive aspects and behaviors that lead to creating a life worth living, your family and friends will notice. A few may even want to join your effort.

In the beginning, this is rough. As you discover how amazing you feel living this way, it will get on your friends' nerves. Really, it will. You will want to share everything you're doing and experiencing. And you will want them to jump on board with you so they can feel as fabulous as you do. When they don't, you'll be prone to judge them. Don't. The rough part is you will watch and be there for them as they continue to live by default and surrender to their adverse conditions, while endlessly complaining about what's going on in their lives. Because of this, you may not want to be around the people you usually hang out with. You may not want to do the things you normally do. As rough as it may be, this is the best thing you can do for yourself.

Be Open

When I talk about transformation, I'm not referring to discovering a new you. I'm referring to discovering the real you, the version of you that existed before the seeds of limited beliefs were planted. These are the beliefs that tell you you're not good enough, you're not pretty enough, you're not young enough, you're not thin enough, you're too thin, you're too tall, or you're too short. I can go on and on about what we think we are not enough of or too much of. Know it is not who you are that holds you back. It is who you think you are not.

You are here to grow and learn from your experiences—the good, the bad, and the ugly. Make good use of what you experience by learning and sharing your wisdom. This knowledge you are acquiring has great value. Wisdom is the foundation of all that we are and all that we do. When you recognize life lessons, grab them and carry them with you. They are valuable. Used well, you will never experience the lesson again, and you can move on to greater things.

You have everything you need right here to make this happen. You can do this. It took me five years because I had to piece everything together. I didn't learn or discover these things as I am sharing them with you here. My journey was complex and convoluted, but I don't want that for you. Take the parts of what I share here that apply to you, and file the rest away for use at another time. Your Flight Plan will take you from where you are now to where you want to be so you can stop walking through life and start flying. When you feel things falling off track, bring yourself back to center and start again. As you take flight, the Spiritual Prescriptions will navigate you through the unchartered skies so you can achieve what you desire.

Honor

Honor your journey by asking for help when you need it from those you trust most. Things don't have to be hard, and you don't have to do this on your own. We all need a hand from time to time.

Having said that, understand that not everyone deserves to hear your story or your struggles, so be selective. Surround yourself with people who love, support, and want the absolute best for you. As you do, you will find supportive people who will inspire you when you are open to receiving them. They will help you get through the muck and pick yourself up when needed.

Commit

Commit to what you want, especially when you feel like crap. To commit is to give trust or charge. When we commit to others, we know what to do. However, when we commit to ourselves, we give up or don't show up with the same energy. We commit to losing weight then overeat as a treat on a Friday night. We commit to improving our lives by choosing to be happy and then throw it all away because it's raining or we didn't get enough attention or there's too much traffic. Time and time again, we betray what we want by giving into chaos and irrationality.

It's time to commit to choosing loving thoughts over fearful thoughts and to move forward, knowing the Infinite Power that moves the energy in this Material World has your back. When you commit, you will not be alone. A whole community is waiting for you at www. WellbeingMessenger.com. They have been where you are. There is no lack of success, and you will never feel lonely or singled out. That's my commitment to you.

Create Time

We don't find time. We create time. If this work is important to you, you will create time to do the work. Do this by focusing on the things that matter at the end of the day when you ask yourself, "Did I show and tell the important people in my life I love them? Did I make a difference and make life a little better? Did I spend my time wisely? Stop spending your time on the path of least resistance, and start investing your time to take the path to your next great adventure. You do this by managing your productivity, not your time.

I'll help you create the time to create your path, but you must make the effort. It will take repeated effort to align your beliefs with your desires and actions. As I've said, this is a practice. If you commit to the practice, as issues arise, you will gain greater clarity and experience more radical shifts that bring more joy and fulfillment into your life. It's amazing and I want you to experience it.

Your commitment to being a Spiritual Girl in a Material World will be challenged. Expect it. Your desires will be disputed by the many responsibilities you have. Your commitment will be challenged by those who love you and need you to do things for them. It will be challenged by your good friend who needs a night off and wants you to go out instead of workout. It will be challenged when you're too tired to do the work. When these things happen, come back. Come back to your center. Connect to your Spiritual Girl.

Life is busy and chaotic. You know this, and that's why you're here. You want to quiet the noise and calm the chaos. Doing this work is a challenge since your day is already bursting at the seams. For you to transform the way you see and experience your world, I need you to honor your desires by investing your time to do the work.

As you move through the components of The Flight Plan, be patient with yourself. There is no judgment, resentment, regret, or anger here. Accept where you are with love. Let go of the fear.

This book is a guide for you to create a life worth living. I cannot tell you what that means; YOU must define what that means. You must discover and declare it for yourself. No one knows what feels good or serves your best interests and highest desires as well as you do. Over the years, you've likely lost your connection to what you want most. I will guide you as you discover your deepest desires, reconnect to your dreams, unlearn the beliefs that hold you back, and uncover all that has been within your reach but that, until now, you did not know how to obtain.

Okay, so we're all set. Are you ready to start moving forward faster? Me too. Let's go!

SPIRITUAL PRESCRIPTION FOR CLARITY

Antidote for feeling lost and stuck in life.

> **I am blessed with absolute clarity, and**
> **my wisdom guides my vision.**

Lack of clarity for what we want is what causes dysfunction in our lives. Clarity gives us purpose. It guides us and gives us a vision of what we are working to achieve.

> **What are you craving in your life?**

Reflection |Connect to the Real You

It's time to find out where you are and how you feel about what is going on in your life. Set aside an hour or so and think about what you feel is missing and what you crave. Then respond to the prompts below.

Be open and honest with yourself. Don't push through them if nothing comes to mind. Seriously ponder them.

Getting clarity on where you want to be will make it easier for you to get there.

> **Each day I feel...**
> **Every day I want to feel...**
> **What are three things I can do to feel**
> **more of what I want to feel?**

Now, it's time for you to fly. Let go, be inspired, and choose happy.

Read your responses with an open heart and mind as you discover were you are not aligned with what you want for yourself. Use these insights to course correct when you stray from your chosen path.

Chapter 4

Live with Passion

*"We cannot solve our problems with the same thinking
we used when we created them." ~Albert Einstein*

Living with Passion means focusing on what brings you joy as you move through your days. When you live with passion, you will naturally foster a more loving and positive perspective of what you view and what you experience.

Living with Passion transforms the way you experience your world, for the better.

You know you need to transform the way you experience your world when you want to experience something different yet continue the patterns that got you to where you didn't want to be. Like when . . .

> You want to stop feeling so exhausted but don't change your habits to improve your eating or sleeping.

> You want to get a higher degree but never enroll in school.

> You want more friends but don't try to connect with new people.

71

You want more love but treat people without regard for their feelings, and you push them away.

You want to feel more supported in your relationships but duck out on your family and friends when the going gets tough and when they need you most.

You are not happy with your life but do nothing to change your circumstances or conditions.

How we think about what we are capable of, who we are, and how we feel about the world impacts our ability to create a life worth living.

Adopt a Thriving Mindset

A Thriving Mindset lifts your self-confidence, giving you the ability to take inspired action to move you farther, faster on the path that leads to health, wealth, and happiness. It empowers you to conquer fears that keep you from your desire to aspire more. A Thriving Mindset deeply connects you to the beliefs and values that serve who you have the full potential of being by creating thoughts that allow you to take inspired action, which propels you toward your dreams, not away from them.

By adopting a Thriving Mindset, you can take one, positive, empowering belief and achieve things you once thought were impossible. You no longer limit yourself to what someone told you when you were ten that led you to believe you were incapable or unworthy of furthering your education, unworthy of getting the career you want, unworthy of finding your soul mate, or unworthy of the money you desired.

I used to say I had a way of surviving, until The Illness. Just surviving put me in bed for nearly a year. That's when I realized that surviving is not good enough for me, and it isn't good enough for you either. It's time to dream a bigger dream, to play a bigger game, to stop walking through life when you can fly.

In this chapter, our goal is to Adopt a Thriving Mindset. When you Adopt a Thriving Mindset, you will challenge your perspective, and you will focus on the thoughts that support you to live with the things that move you: your passions.

A few of the exercises I share to help you create your Flight Plan may seem inconsequential, but I ask that you trust me and do the work anyway. I promise to honor your time and your commitment to creating a life worth living by not wasting your time or energy.

A Thriving Mindset requires you
choose love over fear.

I am not going to debate that feeling good is better than feeling bad and that you deserve to feel good all the time. I am here to be of service to those who know that something is not working in their life and want to find a way to get to a good-feeling place.

Principles of a Thriving Mindset

A Thriving Mindset, what I refer to as Living with Passion, is the first component of The Flight Plan. A Thriving Mindset makes it possible to combat the darkness and heaviness we often experience with fear, and it allows the light of love into our life so we feel more supported in our endeavor to create a life worth living.

We start here because clarity of what you desire through connection to your Inner Guidance is essential preparation for taking on the challenge of calming the chaos, what I refer to as Living with Purpose. There are three Principles of a Thriving Mindset.

Principle 1 | Be mindfully aware. Be mindfully aware of how you feel about your beliefs, thoughts, and actions, and how they affect everything around you.

Principle 2 | Be willing. Be willing to challenge, question, and analyze your emotions and motivations when they do not feel good or right to you.

Principle 3 | Be committed. Be committed to living your life by design and living an authentic, heart-centered lifestyle filled with quality and meaning.

When I discovered these Principles, I was depleted, dismayed, and depressed. By integrating them into my life, I cultivated the wellbeing that connects me to my life and quality living.

Each of the Principles is crucial to developing and maintaining a Thriving Mindset. We are going to dive into them one at a time so you have a full understanding of how to integrate the Principles into your lifestyle.

How You Think Matters

Do you get so caught up in being who you think people want you to be that you forget who you really are?

If so, I want you to know it is absolutely normal in our society, and you are not alone. Most are unaware that there is a good-feeling way to go through life. It's the reason why much of the population has not claimed their wellbeing.

We work too much and play too little. We don't sleep enough and take medications to numb ourselves so we can get through another dissatisfying day. We can't focus on what we need to do and always want to be somewhere other than where we are. This is surviving.

As long as I can remember, I have been a self-help addict. Depression has been a lifelong struggle for me, and from time to time, I still struggle to find peace. All the things I read said, "Let it go and be happy." But I couldn't. I didn't know how. For decades, I spent tens of thousands of dollars on doctors, specialists, pharmaceuticals, and seminars. Yet, that darkness and heaviness would not leave. I did not feel any closer to being the person I knew I had the potential to be.

I had the right tools, but I couldn't figure out how to use them. I didn't want to accept that I couldn't create a fulfilled life, one that felt worth living. I had an incredible career I totally lucked into and was well-respected. I made good money, had a beautiful home, a supportive and loving husband, and three amazing children. Yet, something was missing. I didn't feel whole. I didn't feel satisfied or happy. Keeping it all together was a freaking struggle. I was often closed down, resentful, and rude. These are just a few of the side effects of surviving.

I remember the morning I decided I would no longer own The Illness. I told my family I was done being sick. I told them that from now on, when they asked how I was feeling, I would say, "Great!" no matter how I felt. And no matter what they saw, they were not allowed to treat me as if I was unwell. I instructed them to tell our friends and family I was okay and on the road to health again. I wanted to resuscitate my life. This is how I started my journey to wellness.

I do my best not to pass judgment on others or take part in petty gossip. I no longer watch the news or read newspapers. Whenever I sense negativity or chaos in my space, I work my way through the Thriving Mindset Principles, one by one. More often than not, that keeps me on my path. I have essentially created my very own utopia.

Those who care for me as best they know how have cautioned me. They warn that I'll never know what's going on in the world, I'm not being realistic, and I'm setting myself up for disappointment. I get it. I do. They are trying to protect me. But how does that serve me? I could live in what they say is reality: watching world events, listening to the opinions of others, feeling angry and consumed with the chaos of the Material World, sitting around, worrying about how we are going to make it.

Or, I can focus on what I love, living each moment and enjoying it to the fullest. If things go left when I need them to go right, I deal with it in a manner that honors me and how I want to feel. It doesn't serve me or anyone else to stress out, living in fear about things that could happen.

When we live with a Thriving Mindset and honor how we want to experience life, even when things feel rough and tough, life becomes more effortless. With a Thriving Mindset, life's dramas that normally throw us off a good-feeling path don't gain enough momentum to shift our direction onto a detrimental path that takes us farther from what we want to experience and feel.

Moving Forward – Denise

Denise has worked with me for nine months. She's an amazing doctor who came to me because she was miserable and disliked her work. She became a doctor because no one thought she could do it after getting pregnant in high school. She wanted to prove them wrong. After fifteen years of study and effort, she was working 110 hours a week and hating her life. She had two pre-teen children she felt she did not see enough and hadn't had a serious relationship in over a decade.

As Denise created her Flight Plan, she realized she never forgave herself for giving her daughter up for adoption when she was sixteen. She felt she had to become a doctor to prove to herself that what she sacrificed was justified by her doctor status. She had been in a chain of failed relationships and felt stuck in a life she absolutely hated.

Creating a Flight Plan has empowered Denise to reclaim her personal power and take responsibility for her happiness. She makes different, more empowering, decisions these days. She no long holds on to the guilt or resents the price she paid to go into medicine, and she has forgiven herself for getting pregnant in high school. Today, she works part-time as a doctor so she can enjoy her successes and travel the world, her true passion. She is also opening up to the potential of finding someone to share her newfound time with.

While we have no control over the circumstances that impact our lives, we do have control over how we respond to them.

Ready

As we work our way through the process of creating The Flight Plan, do not judge where you are at this stage of your life, how you got here, or why you made the choices you did. That is not the purpose of our work or time together. Our purpose is to embrace that we are here now, ready, willing, and able to choose differently.

We start here because how you think matters. I can tell you what to do and how to do it, but, until you accept what is possible by getting your mind set, nothing you try will work in the long term.

How you think, your mindset, is your personal power. There are times in our lives when we feel completely powerless. We lose our jobs. We get into accidents. We get sick. Someone we love gets hurt or worse. It's enough to make you wonder why, why you bother living at all.

When you Adopt a Thriving Mindset, you reclaim your personal power by achieving and maintaining full control over your internal feeling state, giving no one and nothing the ability to take it away from you.

Set

I'm going to ask you to be very selfish from here on out. It doesn't mean you do things the way I do them. It means you find ways to do the things that feel good for you from a deep sense of connection and understanding that supports your desired highest and best potential. You may think this is a bad idea. I assure you, if we all lovingly lived more selfishly, this Material World would be what we all know it has the full potential to be.

Imagine having a Thriving Mindset and interacting with the Material World each day, connected to the person you know you have the potential to be, your best and highest loving self. You know—the vision of yourself that shows up at peace, bringing calm to life's chaotic circumstances and noisy situations. Never rattled by the weather, traffic, gossip, or frivolous distractions that most allow to throw their life into utter chaos. Being the ray of sunshine in an otherwise cloudy day, making wise decisions quickly and in alignment with what YOU want. Completely calm and able to respond in a way that honors who you are, leaving behind the frazzled, crazed, unsettled, not-so-loving self when drama ensues.

Go

This is all about getting your "mind set." When we are exhausted and stressed out, we let our emotions and thoughts run rampant, which does not support us or help get us closer to creating what we want to experience in our lives. We must tune up, tap in, and be turned on to get there.

Tune up. Cultivate the mental dexterity to make choices that serve your highest good.

Tap in. Know what serves your highest good.

Turned on. Be aware of what does and does not serve your highest good so you can choose again, when you need to.

When you make a conscious decision to change the way you think, you will find your experiences change for the better without any additional effort. As you take on new actions based on what they MAKE of you, not what they DO for you, the Material World responds in a more supportive way.

Let me share a bit more about each of the Principles. Knowing them and understanding them makes the difference between living by default and living by design.

Principle 1 of a Thriving Mindset | Be Mindfully Aware

The terms "mindful" and "awareness" are ancient, and their meanings have evolved over time. This is a paradox of language. As words become familiar, their original meaning can become vague. The mindfulness movement has blurred the lines as well, and the actual meanings of mindfulness and awareness may be lost. To ensure that we have the same understanding of these terms, I want to clearly define what I'm speaking of when I reference mindfulness and awareness.

Many use mindfulness and awareness interchangeably, but they are notably different. It's important you realize this to understand how each contributes to your wellbeing.

Awareness is knowing what the mind knows—the ability to perceive, to feel, or to be conscious of events, objects, thoughts, emotions, or sensory patterns. In simple terms, it means knowing what is going on.

Awareness is pure observation.

It is the foundation of wellbeing and overcoming the dysfunction of negativity brought on by the chaos of the Material World.

Most of us live in an unconscious manner, playing out the survivor version of our lives and deriving our sense of identity from our misunderstood ego. We tend to label everything around us, which leads to thinking and asking, "What does this mean?" With practice, we learn to allow awareness to guide us to mindfulness, which allows us to change our thinking when necessary and to create the world we want to experience.

Being mindful is having a clear, nonjudgmental understanding of who we are and how we relate to the world, which requires being aware and understanding how our actions affect us and those around us.

Mindfulness is the moment-by-moment awareness of thoughts, feelings, and your surrounding environment. Think of mindfulness as a tool for exploring life experiences. It's a gentle, intuitive way of viewing life, which everyone has the ability to access. Mindfulness can be refined by training and practice.

A 2013 study at the University of California-Santa Barbara found that mindfulness improves reading comprehension, memory capacity, and the ability to focus. University of California-Berkley's Greater Good Center has long studied mindfulness and has found that mindfulness fosters a thriving, resilient, and compassionate society.

In another study on mindfulness (2009), Andrew Olendzki, a classical scholar, stated:

"Like meditation in general, [mindfulness] involves placing attention deliberately upon an object and sustaining it over time unlike [one-pointedness and absorption, another type of meditation] mindfulness tends to open to a broader range of phenomena rather than restricting the focus to a singular object. Like a flood light rather than a spotlight, mindfulness illuminates a more phenomenological field of ever-changing experience rather than isolating a particular object for intensive scrutiny. This alternative mode of observation is necessary because mindfulness practice is more investigating a process than about examining an object."

As Olendzki stated, the development of mindfulness starts with the learning and practice to "place attention deliberately upon an object and sustain it over time." That is, mindfulness starts with awareness.

It sounds simple, right? But given all the complexities of our days, being mindful is challenging. To train ourselves to stop jumping from thought to thought throughout the day, start by focusing on the breath. Listen to the sound of it and keep your attention there for one minute to 20 minutes several times a day.

Mindfulness is directing the mind to direct your thoughts.

Mindful Awareness

Mindfulness and awareness do not refer to how the world relates to us or affects us on a daily basis. Conversely, they relate to our ability to gain a clear, nonjudgmental understanding of who we are and how we relate to the world.

This level of mindful awareness means knowing who you are, what you like, what you believe in, what your values are, what you dislike, how you like to enjoy your "free" time, how you want to be seen by others, and how you want to see yourself. It requires knowing yourself at a profound and meaningful level and understanding how this self-knowing affects you and those around you.

Awareness is knowing where you are.
Mindfulness is knowing how you got there.

We become mindfully aware so we can take responsibility for how our personality, emotions, and behaviors affect us and those around us.

For instance, when you work at your desk for a couple of hours, and you suddenly notice you have a headache, awareness has helped you recognize you have a headache. Mindfulness is careful attention to how you got the headache. Each plays its part, leading you on the path to finding a solution to what ails you, which may be popping a pill, drinking several cups of water, or taking a three-minute breathing/meditation break.

Knowing yourself at this intimate level leaves you unshaken by opinions and persuasions. This empowers you to act from a deep sense of knowing what it is that will most serve your highest good without question, so you are not swayed by The Others.

After years, or perhaps even decades, of being who we think we are supposed to be, many of us are no longer connected to what makes our hearts flutter or our stomachs flip in joy. Without taking stock of our own sense of fulfillment, we sometimes find ourselves on the path of least resistance, even when it feels all wrong. It shouldn't come as a surprise when we feel completely empty and lost. But, for most of us, it does.

What does adopting a Thriving Mindset look like in everyday life?

We are about to explore how to make positive changes in the way you think so you no longer feel pressured to do and be everything. Adopting a Thriving Mindset that embraces health, wealth, and happiness makes it easier to do away with the notion that we must achieve perfection.

When you cultivate mindful awareness in your life, you get to know yourself in a way you never experienced before. It really is awe-inspiring, because when you understand yourself better, you:

> Gain more control over how you show up in all situations so nothing triggers emotional responses; you are able to react in a manner that honors you and the way you want to live.

Go with the flow of life when you face challenges; you show up fully engaged and ready to find a solution rather than dwell on the problem.

Feel confident knowing you are empowered with the ability to take inspired steps on your path to passion, purpose, and play by reframing negative thoughts and emphasizing positive ones.

Respond to everything in your life in alignment with your beliefs and core values in the forefront, so you never feel betrayed by your thoughts, and you never turn your back on the essence of who you really are.

Improve your connections, communication, and understanding in your relationships, allowing them to deepen and be more meaningful.

Make good decisions that strengthen your commitment to living well, so you never feel like life is running you, and you always feel like an active participant in your life.

Clearly understand your feelings, beliefs, and thoughts, so you get the upper hand when you're up against life's toughest situations.

By knowing our strengths and weaknesses and by taking actions to account for them, we are more effective in dealing with life's everyday chaos of the Material World, and we can more deliberately create a life worth living.

Imagine what your life will look like when you master mindful awareness. Imagine being so present that you learn from your experiences. Instead of being the victim, you become the victor, because you are able to extract the golden nuggets from your lessons. These golden nuggets are the gifts that empower you to choose differently so you experience more of what you want and less of what you don't want.

*   *   *

Understanding yourself at a deep level gives you the ability to recognize which habits you can cultivate to improve how you feel and enhance your quality of life. Being mindfully aware gives you a broader perspective on the way we interact with ourselves and others.

SPIRITUAL PRESCRIPTION FOR MINDFUL AWARENESS

Antidote for lack of joy, gratitude, and happiness, when you feel disconnection and lack excitement for your experiences.

I am the master of my thoughts and beliefs.

When you feel disconnected and don't know where to start, start here.

A Spiritual Girl knows her feelings are indicators of how well she is living in alignment. By giving attention to how she feels, she can counteract her defaulted, limiting beliefs and thoughts; this is essential when the chaos and noise of the Material World block out any intentions she has set about how she wants to feel and think as she goes through her day.

Cultivate Mindful Awareness

There are two simple ways to cultivate Mindful Awareness.

First, be present during daily experiences.

Treat life like a classroom. Learn from your mistakes. Be in observance, not judgment, of them. Carry the wisdom extracted from your lessons to stop unpleasant cycles from repeating themselves.

Second, get to know yourself at a deeper level.

Get curious about yourself and ask questions. What colors do you like? What makes you come alive? What do you suck at and what do you do well? What do you enjoy doing and don't enjoy doing? Dive deep. You never know what you will discover about yourself.

Reflection | Better-Feeling Days

As we move through our days, we don't pay attention, which is why things get out of control. We live on auto-pilot. This is a simple but powerful exercise. It will tell you so much about how you think and feel by default each day. It will help you give attention to how you feel physically and emotionally, about your actions, beliefs, and thoughts.

Do the following at the beginning, the middle, and the end of your day, three times a day.

Get yourself into a relaxed state by taking a few deep breaths. Ask yourself:

How am I feeling?

Take deep breaths until you feel calm and relaxed. Give careful attention to your emotional state and corresponding bodily sensations as they respond to your question.

Write your observations and thoughts.

Set a reminder to do this at 7 a.m., 4 p.m., and 9 p.m. or generally in these intervals, as your schedule permits.

As you go through the exercise, do not judge yourself. Give attention to your physical sensations and emotions. They are instruments and respond to your actions, beliefs, and thoughts throughout your day. There is no right or wrong here, no good or bad. Only high vibe and low vibe.

If you discover you are low vibe, this is an opportunity to consider things you could do differently so you feel high vibe more often.

If you discover you are high vibe, excellent. Keep doing those things that make you feel fulfilled and good.

Principle 2 of a Thriving Mindset | Be Willing

Cultivating willingness allows us to be more open to expansive discovery. When you are willing to learn, to mentally and emotionally challenge the thoughts and beliefs that don't serve your best interests, you uncover solutions to make yourself invincible to life's setbacks. Creating a life worth living becomes not simply possible but probable.

Imagine what life will be like when all your false and limiting beliefs disappear, leaving a blank slate where endless possibilities become valid options for living, and nothing holds you back from being or doing everything you want. Wouldn't that be freaking amazing? You can have that.

Our actions are driven by our thoughts, which are driven by our beliefs. This is why it's so important to be willing to examine our beliefs. We don't want to end up living far below our true desired potential and never achieve what we are fully capable of achieving. When we are unwilling, and closed to new ways of doing and thinking, we block our potential to achieve higher levels of wellbeing.

Our negative and positive life experiences are the consequences of our actions.

Beliefs

A belief is a thought we regard as truth—either about ourselves or others, or the way the world works. However, our beliefs do not always reflect reality.

For instance, when we believed the world was flat, we thought we would fall off the edge of the earth if we sailed far enough. Today, we know that's not true. The flat earth theory is a good example of how our beliefs can be utterly false.

Our beliefs fuel our actions, behaviors, emotions, and motivations. They play a significant role in our personal development and influence the level of success we feel is possible. When we don't have strong, supportive beliefs about ourselves, we diminish our self-worth and, hence, are prohibited from learning what we are capable of and realizing our full potential.

Our beliefs are a direct result of our daily experiences, our interactions with our family and friends, and judgments by others and ourselves. The level of success we achieve, the failures we experience, and our religious beliefs are all factors that govern what we accept and reject.

Your beliefs determine the course of your life more than any other influence, so attention must be given. The things you have achieved or failed to achieve in your life are a direct result of your beliefs.

You can only transform your life when you are willing to question why you are the person you are. It is critical to accept the possibility that many beliefs you regard to be true may actually be false.

Influencers

Our upbringing, the media, our friends, and society influence the types of beliefs and values we live by. We model our behavior after those who are closest to us. In our childhood, it's our family members. They tell us what is good and bad. We learn to act a certain way, and we create beliefs about how and who we should be.

It is estimated we receive over 3,000 messages and images each day, telling us how to be, what to do, and why we should do it. These can confuse us and throw us off our desired path. They can change what we think and how we act while we strive to carry out our purpose of creating a life we love. If we want it to be filled with belonging, connection, ease, and joy, we need to do away with the fears, resentment, judgments, and anger these messages and images sometimes foster in us.

We accept behaviors based on what we see, which is not always in alignment with our values. We choose friends who we think we should be like and who we look to for approval. Understand that certain people are in your life for a reason. Some, both friends and family members, will come and go because of life circumstances. When that happens, we must accept and release them without fear or judgment.

A Spiritual Girl must always give attention to how influences make her feel. This guides her to make decisions in alignment with her best interests and highest desired potential.

Willpower

Despite having limiting beliefs, some people still move forward. They achieve what they want through sheer determination and willpower, making things feel harder than they need to feel. The problem with willpower is that when you're exhausted and stressed out, you simply don't have it to give.

Rather than using willpower, be willing. Willingness empowers you to do things you never thought possible: to discover your passions in life and disprove fears so you can dream and achieve big things. Let go of the façade and live authentically; show up open, ready, and willing at your absolute best-feeling self.

As we release our death grip on our fears and limiting beliefs, we reclaim our enthusiasm and excitement to create a lifestyle to which we are fully engaged and connected. To improve our lives, we must be willing to transform the beliefs that do not empower us, do not feel good, and do not resonate with us any longer. An easy way to expand is to question what you believe and do your own research so you can make informed decisions about what is true and feels good for you.

Understand that your truth, or your version of the truth, is entirely based on your perspective and how you interpret things. Your truth is likely not the same as someone else's truth. Don't accept everything that appears true at face value. When something seems true, find information to support that belief before you accept it as truth.

Reframing

Do you ever think, I am stuck and have no options? Who do I think I am to want to be better?

If someone spoke to you the way you speak to yourself, would you be friends? Probably not. However, most of us continue negative dialogues that keep us from dreaming bigger dreams for ourselves. Living small serves no one. That little voice keeps us from growing and discovering our passion and true potential.

We have between 50,000 and 70,000 thoughts each day. That's 35 to 48 thoughts every minute.

Isn't that amazing?

Our beliefs fuel our thoughts, our thoughts fuel the emotions we experience, and our emotions fuel the actions we carry out. Our beliefs are critical to our health, wealth, and happiness. They dictate the way we interact with people and how we feel about the world, which can make the difference between surviving and thriving. As the years pass and as we learn and grow, it's important to question our beliefs when they don't feel right.

A technique called "reframing" allows us to identify those attacking thoughts that come from sabotaging beliefs and to replace them with more positive and empowering ones. You can literally reframe in a positive manner any belief that doesn't serve you.

As you reframe beliefs that don't serve you, keep these three things in mind.

Don't assign meaning to events or situations.

We assign labels and meaning to events and situations based on our own perceptions. Refrain from constantly thinking, "What does this mean to me?" Instead, simply be in the moment and enjoy the experience for what it is.

We miss many things when we live on automatic pilot. Being present, by focusing on the moment-by-moment activity that surrounds you, will provide the opportunity to marvel at the miracles of life instead of taking them for granted.

Don't believe everything you think.

One day, I was doing laundry and realized the twins were a few minutes late coming home from school. At the time, they were sophomores in high school and took the school bus that left them about a block from the house. My mind went on a rampage about all the things that could have happened.

The bus could have been in an accident.

Roque could have gotten into a fight on the bus.

They could have walked home instead, and a car could have hit them.

Then I stopped myself. I realized that just because I think it, I don't have to respond to it. I can choose to think differently.

This was the first time in my life I realized that I don't have to believe everything I think.

I wish our crazy thoughts were easy to deal with. But we face much more difficult and detrimental thoughts daily than I describe here. Your thoughts stem from a belief that you can choose to ignore so they don't impact how you feel, especially when they have no basis in fact.

Don't dismiss your "bad" thoughts.

Thoughts that you keep thinking, repetitively, deserve your attention; understanding where they come from will help.

When you notice a pattern of thinking you don't enjoy, it's time to challenge the belief those thoughts stem from. In the Spiritual Prescription for Willingness, I walk you through a process I created as the antidote for being rigid, inflexible, and closed off to new and revised beliefs that support you. It allows you to reflect on your beliefs in a way that honors you and how you want to feel.

Before we continue, this is a good time to take on "bad" and "good" versus "like" and "hate." Words have power, so we should heed how we use them. In an effort to avoid labeling things, I try not to refer to emotions as being good or bad, and I avoid saying I like or hate things. Now I say I feel heavy or low instead of bad. I say I feel light and high vibe when I feel good. I also changed the way I refer to what I dislike by saying it is not an energetic match.

Words are powerful, and we must use care in choosing the words we say to ourselves and others. Once spoken, words cannot be forgotten, only forgiven.

SPIRITUAL PRESCRIPTION FOR WILLINGNESS

Antidote for unsupportive thoughts that keep you stuck in patterns that do not support your potential.

I am willing to do what is required to create a life I love.

A limiting belief is a belief you keep thinking that does not support what you want for yourself, and keeps or limits you from doing something you want to do or going after something you want to have or experience.

A Spiritual Girl deals with those pesky, unsupportive beliefs and thoughts that don't help her feel the way she wants to feel by reframing the beliefs and thoughts that keep her from living out loud and enjoying all the things that are speaking to her soul.

Reflection | Reign in Unsupportive Beliefs

Are you willing to question your beliefs?

These steps will empower you to move forward and grow beyond the boundaries you set for yourself. You will discover that many of the beliefs holding you back are false, have no basis, and thus, can be rejected.

Once you are aware something is false, being mindful will slow your thought process. Then, your reactions will start to change to accommodate your new empowering belief. This process will occur more rapidly the more times you disprove the original belief.

Relieve stress and pressure by releasing beliefs that keep you stuck.

Step 1 | *Observe your thoughts.*

To observe your thoughts and feel your energy shift, you must be fully present and mindfully aware. If you sense a negative feeling come up with a thought, pay attention to it by writing it down.

Recording it serves a couple of purposes. First, it immediately stops the flow of negative thought. Second, you learn about yourself when you journal your thoughts. You will see what your thoughts naturally default to, which is powerful when intending to transform the way you experience the Material World.

As you practice this, you will be able to rationalize your feelings and more easily respond rather than react. Your response can be presented without any sense of fear, showing up as impatience, intolerance, jealousy, resentment, or anger. You will be able to keep a calm head in the times of chaos. As a result, you will have much better and stronger relationships.

Some people put a rubber band around their wrist and snap it when they have a belief they want to reframe. This is a good practice when you are creating new habits. The rubber band serves as your reminder of who you are and how you want to be. I use a mala bead wrap bracelet for this. It's a beautiful constant reminder of my commitment to creating a life worth living, and it's much gentler than a rubber band.

This first step is critical when seeking to overcome limiting thoughts that don't allow you to step fully into the person you know you have the potential to be.

Step 2 | *Replace an unsupportive thought with a positive one.*

There are several ways to replace negative thoughts with positive thoughts.

Think from a place of love. This is a creative, fun method for reframing your beliefs. Thinking from a place of love means using high-vibe thoughts and words to empower you. This is the easiest and fastest way to reframe a negative thought.

Do away with assumptions. When you have a recurring thought that doesn't feel good, it likely comes from a limiting belief. Limiting beliefs keep you stuck in your situation. A limiting belief is usually based on assumptions that you have drawn from your experiences or the experiences of others.

When you notice a limiting belief or thought arise, write down all the reasons your belief is not true. Rationalizing and working through limiting beliefs keeps them from getting the better of you.

If a limiting belief comes up consistently, you can go a bit further with it.

Begin to rationalize your thoughts by asking yourself:

What am I supposed to learn from this?
Where did this come from?
Is it true?
Does this serve my best interest?
What better-feeling thought can I create from this?

Often, unsupportive thoughts recur in our lives when we haven't yet accepted a life lesson.

As the spectators of our lives, we witness how people allow chaos into theirs. You can clearly see the cycles, but they usually do not. This happens in reverse as well. However, in the middle of chaos, the repetitive cycles are not easily noticeable. Being observant of our thoughts gives us the necessary perspective to hone in on our patterns of disaster so we can shift them to something more empowering and better-feeling.

Certain situations may come up over and over in your life. You may play them out time after time in mini-melodramas with different casts of characters. Until, finally, you get it. And make no mistake. You. Will. Get. It. *When* is up to you and is determined by how well you pay attention to the signs.

Addressing these beliefs and thoughts one at a time will empower you to take on those bigger challenges.

One by one, reframe each belief and thought, either until you feel good about the statement or, at the very least, until it is neutral. Track these thoughts by writing them in a notebook as they arise. At the end of the day, review your list and reframe them.

Principle 3 of a Thriving Mindset | Be Committed

Are you committed to living your life by your design
and no longer allowing the noise and distraction of
daily life to force you into living by default?

Being committed is a pledge to a position on an issue or a question.

When we commit to others, we understand what is involved:

Being where you say you will be when you say you will be there.

Being prepared and arming yourself with the right tools to get the job done.

Doing what you say you are going to do when you say you are going to do it.

Showing courage and strength to achieve your desired outcomes.

Applying concentrated effort to your tasks.

Never giving up! Ever!!!

Springing back with ease and getting back to the task at hand when setbacks are encountered.

Right?

However, when we commit to ourselves, we don't show up in the same light. We lack energy and enthusiasm about our commitments to ourselves when it comes time to achieve our deepest desires. We promise we will exercise and eat better, but we fold under pressure on a Friday night after a long week. We wake up feeling like walking zombies and promise ourselves we will sleep more, but we continue to sleep only four to six hours a night, knowing we need eight.

How do you commit to a Thriving Mindset?

In the following pages, I will share how a Spiritual Girl commits to living a life by design, so you can cultivate a Thriving Mindset about your life circumstances and experiences. This will help you choose love over fear so you make decisions that support your highest potential to create a life worth living. When we make decisions in tune with our Thriving Mindset and act from that place of pure, positive inspiration, life flows more effortlessly.

Achieving and maintaining a Thriving Mindset is a life-long practice you must be committed to. Being aware, being willing, and being committed are just the beginning to transforming the way you experience your world.

Choose Love Over Fear

During my challenges with depression, I used prescribed medications to help manage my symptoms. While I have chosen not to take medication since 2012, I still struggle periodically with that deep, hollow weight of depression for reasons I don't understand. I know I'm not alone.

Millions upon millions of people out there also struggle with depression and the symptoms related to it. Readers of my blog who are experiencing depression right now may be triggered by what I am about to say, but I have to say it because I know it to be true. So please, allow me to apologize in advance. I say this with love and to be of service.

You can choose in every millisecond how you feel and reach for a higher feeling when you are feeling down, or low-vibe. Stay with me here, please. Practically, it goes something like this.

The morning I wrote this for you, this was my thinking:

On October 30, 2013, my Abuella transitioned. Every fall since then, I have a lot of emotional and physical issues from the amount of grief I feel. Grief is one of the lowest emotions we can experience. I sat down one day to write about my feelings and cried a bit. Then I posted an entry on Facebook about what I learned from her. Someone commented on my post that every time I remember my Abuella, her love is reignited in the world. That comment left me feeling so hopeful. It immediately lifted my spirit and gave me the energy to continue writing this for you. I became filled with gratitude for having my Abuella in my life at all, one of the highest emotional states we can achieve.

What I realize today that I did not realize before is when I struggle with depression I can reach for the next, higher-feeling emotion. I don't have to stay stuck at the bottom, and neither do you.

Please don't misunderstand me. Do I think you can go from feeling depression to joy in a matter of minutes? No, I don't. I have been practicing and making a choice to feel better for over five years and continue to do so today.

If you are thinking, "It's not easy to cultivate happiness and choose love," I agree with you. But I'll also tell you that it doesn't mean it's not possible. For those who say, "Carmen, I just feel so stuck, sad, and heavy. I cannot deal with it," my response is, "You are not looking inward for your happiness. You are looking outward."

If this describes any of what you are feeling, I am happy and incredibly grateful you are here. By the time you finish this book, you are not only going to feel unstuck and unburdened, but you will also feel hopeful and inspired.

Another book I read as I began my recovery from neurological Lyme disease, which had left me clinically depressed, depleted and disabled, helped me with my longtime struggle and feelings of victimhood. The book is called ***Ask and It Is Given***, by Esther and Jerry Hicks.

The book shares an *Emotional Guidance Scale* that goes like this:

High-Vibe Feelings
1. Joy / Knowledge / Empowerment / Freedom / Appreciation / Love
2. Passion
3. Enthusiasm
4. Positive Expectation Belief
5. Optimism
6. Hopefulness
7. Contentment

Lower Vibe Feelings
8. Boredom
9. Pessimism
10. Frustration / Irritation / Impatience
11. Overwhelm
12. Disappointment
13. Doubt
14. Worry
15. Blame
16. Discouragement
17. Anger
18. Revenge
19. Hatred / Rage

20. Jealousy
21. Insecurity / Guilt / Unworthiness
22. Fear / Grief / Depression / Powerlessness / Victim

Now that we know we have a choice in how we feel each day, our job to reach for the next higher feeling, until we get to the top, just got easier.

A Spiritual Girl makes a conscious choice every minute of every day about how she feels. It is not something you do once. It takes practice, and it's abso-freaking-lutely worth it.

When a situation drags you down, and you're feeling heavy and low vibe, here's how to choose love and reach for that higher feeling.

How to Choose Love and Reach for That Higher Feeling

Step 1 |Take a deep breath. Taking a deep breath brings in new oxygen, which helps your brain and body function better. When you feel a "bad" or lower emotion come on, deal with it by taking a deep breath.

Step 2 | Respond in your time. Don't react to things, circumstances, and situations in the way you always have. Our old patterns are deeply ingrained, so be patient with yourself. To experience true transformation, we must release old thought patterns that do not serve us and create new patterns that empower us.

Step 3 | Process all your options. We always have a choice, and we must take responsibility for the choices we make. Do you choose to react or to respond? You may ask, what's the difference? When you react to something, you act reciprocally upon the situation or person. When you respond to something, you act favorably to the situation or individual.

Step 4: | *Move forward in alignment.* Look at situations from your highest and best intentions to find your best options. Consider:

Which actions empower you?
Which actions feel good to you?
Which actions honor you?

Step 5 | *Reach up.* After you've taken that deep breath and a moment to consider your options, you can start to resolve lower feelings and select higher, better feelings about your situation.

Next time you wake up or something happens that takes you off your good-feeling path, remember that you have a choice to move up. You don't find joy; you create it.

So instead of thinking...

"It's raining, so today is going to be nasty and messy. My pants are going to get dirty walking from the train station to work, and I'm going to get soaked," think, "Okay, it's raining. I'll wear a skirt and my hair in a ponytail, so I don't have to worry about my clothes. I'll take a taxi from the station to work, so I don't get wet. What a sweet treat."

Or rather than thinking...

"It's so cold today. I hate dressing up in all those thick, heavy clothes. Why can't it be 80 degrees every day?" think, "It's a crisp day. Let me pull out my cozy turtlenecks and scarves. I love that snug, warm feeling my clothes give me on these chilly days."

Or instead of thinking...

"Wow, there are a lot of cars out here. I can't believe how slow everyone is going. Damn, if only I could get in that lane where they're going a little faster," think, "So many people are looking to get to where they're going. Let me turn on my tunes and sing my butt off to my jams. It's a beautiful day. I'm lucky to spend a little more time out here."

It's that simple to choose love over fear.

Moving Forward – Molly

Molly is a real estate agent who has been in business for over 20 years. She was widowed when the eldest of her three children was 7 and the youngest 2. We have been working together for three months.

When Molly found me, she was craving stronger relationships in her life. Financially, she does well for herself, but now in her 40s, she has felt her life to be incomplete. She wants a companion to share her life with and to get to know her kids again. She is often stressed out and, by her own admission, a bit rough in how she speaks to her family, children, and clients. She doesn't enjoy being "hard" all the time, but feels no one will take her seriously if she's not. After overhearing a conversation her children were having about how difficult and unhappy she was, Molly realized something had to change. That's not the way she wants to be spoken about or remembered.

I asked her how she wants people to describe her. She said loving, independent, and strong. Together, we defined what each of these words means to her. Then we set up two daily reminders so she can check in with her words and, if necessary, reconcile her behavior with how she wants people to describe and experience her.

Since defining and focusing on how she wants people to describe her, Molly says she has been more careful and caring with her words. After a couple of weeks, her eldest son, now 17, told her she seems less stressed and nicer. She was so excited she started to cry because that's exactly what she wanted.

Today, Molly has new words: enthusiastic, joyous, and loving. She also has a newfound companion. Molly says when she realized she can reflect what she wants people to remember about her, everything changed. She thought she was doomed to live out her years unfulfilled and incomplete. She now realizes she has a choice in how she is remembered, and her words remind her how she wants to be and interact with others.

The Behaviors

There are seven stand-out behaviors we can cultivate to create a life worth living and by our design. These behaviors are practiced by those who have already mastered their wellbeing and achieved success.

Behavior 1 | Be Present

Being present means existing or occurring now. Dwelling on the *should haves* and *could haves*, or the best and worst of times, prevents us from fully embracing what we have in this moment.

The type of presence I am talking about cultivating means leaving the past behind you and the future to the fortune tellers. It allows you to be grateful and understand what you are experiencing and why. Your misery or happiness wholly depends on your attitude in each moment.

When you can find the good in your experiences, the more good you will experience.

Look for the good in your daily experiences. They are there. I promise they are.

Behavior 2 | Be Tuned In

Being Tuned In is my ritual for centering and returning to love throughout the day. I Tune In at the beginning and the end of the day and between major tasks. This process helps ignite a Thriving Mindset.

The purpose of Tuning In is to bring yourself to center when you feel off-centered, for whatever reason. Before you start working on your Spiritual Prescriptions, Tune In so you can find your center no matter what is going on in the Material World. This will empower your inner Spiritual Girl to release any frustration, overwhelm, and stress that builds up, and help you embrace the calm and flow that makes life feel better.

Tuning In is your gateway to doing what you want when you want to do it so you never feel stuck or struggle with what to do next.

I am sharing my Tuning In Process as a starting point. Use this when you need to get inspired and motivated to do the work.

Let's face it, we can plan and schedule and still, things don't always come together when it's time. This Tune In Process will give you the edge you need to honor your commitment.

Tune In Process

Breathe. Take a series of deep breaths. Inhale and exhale as you feel comfortable. Do this until you feel relaxed. This boost of oxygen will increase your brain power and signal to your body it is time to return to center.

Get set. Think about why you are taking this time to focus. It is your reason for the action you are taking. This helps you prepare to act with enthusiasm. Ask yourself, "Why do I want to do this? What will it help me achieve? How will it get me closer to the success I crave?"

Next, make an affirmative statement to help you get into a positive state.

My Get Set Affirmative Statement

I am working on (state the work you are about to do)
for the next (the intended amount of time you will work on your project),
so I can make my dreams a reality and achieve my goals.
During this time, I will be open to guidance.
I am reclaiming my time and calming the chaos
so I may transform the way I experience my world
and achieve the success I desire without sacrificing
my health, wealth, and happiness.

Set the mood. Set yourself up for success by setting the mood. From how you dress to the environment you sit in, consider what you want to do and how you want to feel while doing it. Then do what feels good.

Sometimes I play music, light a candle, drink tea, or go for a walk. Do what feels calming to you while holding your intention to take focused, inspired action.

Engage your body. Stand up and bounce on your toes. This really soothes the neck and shoulder muscles. Do this for a minute and a half while breathing deeply. You may also want to stretch your neck and extend your arms. This will help release any nervous energy and resistance you may have regarding the work at hand.

Prepare. Design your space to support your success. Set up your creation station so, when you are ready to go, you don't have to look for anything. This will help you stay focused.

Breathe again. Settle into your chair. Take a series of deep breaths. Do this until you feel completely relaxed and all thoughts about anything other than what you are going to work on have dissipated.

Do the work. You are ready for success. Get to work. Stay in the present moment and enjoy the flow. Honor your commitment to your desires.

This process takes about five minutes. Use the Tuning In Process whenever you want to focus your energy. If you find thoughts bubbling up throughout your Tune In Process, that's fine. Acknowledge them and write down anything you want to remember. Then let them go.

If you enjoy this Tuning In Process, excellent! Use it. If it doesn't resonate with you or you still have trouble focusing, modify it or create a process that works for you.

Behavior 3 | Be Inspired

Taking focused, inspired action that supports who you are and how you want to feel with conviction and clarity makes achieving the impossible possible. We all have the power to accomplish anything we want when we set our minds. Yes, I know that's what people have told you for decades, but until now, no one has told you how.

Imagine you decide to make a dream reality. You commit to that dream, making it a goal. Then, you act to make it happen. While acting and working your mojo, you knock tasks off your to-do list two at a time at lightning speed. Within a couple of weeks, working through objections and what seemed like insurmountable barriers, you run out of steam. At a dead stop, your energy depleted, you decide to shelf your project. Your dream will have to wait to see the light of day. Now I ask you, "Are you motivated or inspired?"

Inspiration v. Motivation

Being inspired arises from an inexplicable inner calling. Being motivated comes from a notion of obligation.

Inspiration comes from a feeling deep inside when you are called to do something. The word inspiration means to be in spirit. Inspiration carries you through the process of transforming your deepest desires into reality. When you're inspired, you feel perfectly aligned and natural as you take action toward achieving your goals.

Motivation comes from feeling that you should do something, without thinking or considering why. It requires much more willpower as you manage your to-do list, and exhaustion and worry inevitably take over. When you are motivated, you feel your challenges are innumerable.

When you act from an inspired place, everything falls into place. Your thoughts and actions are perfectly aligned toward the same goal. When you are motivated, you'll notice that feelings of exhaustion, worry, and overwhelm take over, making it difficult to focus, making every effort and action you take feel like a waste of time.

Inspiration drives you and permeates your inner being, helping you gain momentum with ease. Motivation compels us, but at the end of the day, it does not keep our momentum going. Then, feelings of doubt creep in and take over. This is how you know you have moved out of inspiration and into motivation.

It may feel impossible to be in an inspired state in every moment. However, being mindfully aware, you can catch yourself quickly when you move out of alignment and stray from your intended path. If you feel frantic and depleted, you are in motivation mode. If you feel self-assured and excited, you have moved into an inspired mode.

I am all about effortlessness and making things as easy as possible. I have found a few ways to keep my inner Spiritual Girl inspired while the Material World relentlessly tries to knock the wind out of her. My Peace Practice is one of them.

Peace Practice

Each day, crappy things happen and sometimes you need a little help managing the emotions and feelings that arise. This is when we go to our Peace Practice. A Peace Practice includes a combination of focusing on an affirmation, journaling, meditation, and visualization.

A Peace Practice enables you to focus on who you are so you show up in the Material World connected to your best and highest self. Do it at the beginning of each day. If your life is absolutely nuts and you feel out of control, do it twice, once at the beginning and once at the end.

Journal
Your Peace Practice begins with journaling.

Use your journal to capture your thoughts. Over time, these thoughts will become calls for action. Through journaling, you will discover your deepest thoughts, which allows you to explore them.

This practice is not about creating a diary about all things that went wrong in your day. This practice is about looking at something that you experienced and how it unfolded. If it is a good highlight of your day, celebrate it. If it wasn't, look to see how it could have played out differently in a positive way. It is imperative to focus on what you specifically could change, when appropriate, to achieve better outcomes. Remember, we cannot control other people, only ourselves, so our solutions must include action steps we can take on our own.

Each day, I start journaling by writing the date, the day, and, in a few words, how I generally feel. Then, I note any significant issues or imbalances. For each problem I write about, I commit to finding a solution.

Journaling has been critical to transforming how I interpret things in my life. Before I make changes to my life on the outside, I do a lot of work inside. As I do, much of my outside world transforms with little effort on my part.

When you journal during your Peace Practice, it's important to integrate actions that strengthen your commitment to living in alignment. Each day, record the feelings and situations that stood out. When you are feeling unwell, this is a good place to look for what could be the underlying cause of any angst.

Meditation
After you clear your thoughts, meditate.

Meditation is the single, most powerful behavior you can adopt to increase your health, wealth, and happiness. Deepak Chopra says mediation gives us that critical millisecond between our thoughts to consider the way we think, which gives us an opportunity to be responsive in a way that is in alignment with our highest and best selves.

Until a few years ago, I thought I had to follow every thought I had. Meditation helped me realize I can pick and choose the thoughts I give attention and momentum to and dismiss the rest. Talk about empowering! Meditation also helps sooth pain and calm anxieties when they show up.

Meditation can lessen worry, anxiety, and impulsivity, as well as reduce stress, fear, loneliness, and depression. Meditation enhances self-esteem and self-acceptance and increases optimism, relaxation, and awareness. Meditation also helps prevent emotional eating and smoking. It helps develop positive social connections and improves mood and emotional intelligence. All the benefits have profound effects on our wellbeing.

Meditation benefits our minds by boosting mental strength and focus, increasing memory retention and recall, and improving cognitive skills and creative thinking. People who meditate have better decision-making and problem-solving skills. They process information better and ignore distractions.

Last, but not least, meditation contributes to a healthy body by improving our immune system and energy levels, improving breathing and heart rates, and reducing blood pressure. It improves longevity, lessens heart and brain problems, decreases inflammatory disorders and asthma, and diminishes premenstrual and menopausal syndromes. It even helps prevent arthritis and fibromyalgia.

Affirmation
Set your personal intention through affirmation.

An affirmation is anything you say or think. What we want to focus on are positive affirmations. As you get started with affirmations, it's important to put yourself in a state where you can believe your affirmation is or can be true. You must get yourself to a good-feeling place, which is why we meditate before affirmations. Allow yourself the emotions that come through your experiences. Don't judge them. Don't be ashamed of them. You matter and how you feel matters. Honor that by letting the energy of that emotion flow. When we do this, we stop getting stuck and holding ourselves back. Through this energy of flow, we can generate feelings we want to experience through affirmations.

Affirmations mark the beginning point for transformation. Choose words that will empower you to eliminate something from your life or help you create something new in your life. Start doing this by speaking about what you want and stop talking about what you don't want.

When you transform the way you think, everything in your life transforms. You will be amazed at how you begin to experience the Material World when you change your thoughts with affirmations.

If you continuously say to yourself, "I hate my body," instead, say, "I desire to love and appreciate my body."

If you say, "I never have money for what I want," instead say, "I desire money to flow easily and frequently into my life."

If you say, "I am sick and tired of being sick and tired," instead say, "I desire my body to return to its natural, healthy state."

Don't obsess about every thought you have, but as you begin the transformation, notice them. When you catch a negative thought, stop it. Remind yourself that the thought is an old one, and say to yourself, "I choose to think differently." Then, find a positive thought to replace that old thought.

The goal is to feel as good as you can, as often as you can.

Behavior 4 | Be Aligned

Living in alignment with your desires is the key to creating a life worth living.

Looking to transcend and achieve something "more" is a natural desire that resides in each of us. What we want is always changing based on our current state of connection with who we are and, as we evolve, through our experiences. It takes time, dedication, and daily practice to live in alignment with what we desire most.

When I speak about alignment, I mean aligning with your higher loving self, aligning with your best interests, aligning with what you truly desire: that version of yourself you know you are meant to be but are not yet because of fear—fear of what others will think, fear for how things around you will change, fear that you will be an outcast, fear that you will fail. When you know what you want to feel, align your actions with clarity of what you desire so you can experience supportive emotions.

Alignment is honoring your higher loving self to do the things that you say you want to do.

Living in alignment means bringing the important components of your life into proper or desirable coordination and correlation. When you get this right, life flows more effortlessly and you feel more joyous.

Stop giving your dreams lip service and start giving them due service.

If you want to feel the pride of home ownership and don't own one, you may have to work harder, find a new job, or a second job to make more money. Even though you don't want to work more, focusing on your goal of a new home gives you the inspiration to keep going when the going gets rough.

Create more flow in your life by bringing yourself into full alignment. Align your beliefs, thoughts, and actions with what you truly desire: your dreams.

How do you know when you are aligned?

Here are signs of being aligned.

Feeling more optimistic.

Feeling compelled to try new things.

Finding what you desire with more ease.

Feeling joyous more often, for no reason.

Having what you need to do the things you want.

Being more conscious about eating healthy foods.

The desire to relax and simply be, more than ever before.

Having fantastic ideas for yourself and others.

Tiring of the busyness and wanting more meaning in your life.

Newfound desire to seek out adventure and exploration.

Pointing out everyday beauty to others, such as birds flying.

Feeling gratitude for things that are commonplace, such as trees and electricity.

Seeking more nurturing activities such as baths, massages, and body healing.

Attracting people similar to you when you are at your high, feeling your best, and reaching for your full potential.

Finding the courage to live from a place of love and sharing that love with others, when you would otherwise keep it to yourself.

Imagine with me for a moment that you work 50 hours a week and spend an additional 10 hours commuting. You cook, clean, and care for the significant people in your life. You are so exhausted that when you get a moment to yourself all you want to do is plop in front of the television.

You know you need to calm your chaos. You seek clarity about what you want so you can find the solutions to make things better. Do you want to do more meaningful work? Do you want help from the people you live with so you can stop feeling crushed under the weight of your responsibilities? Do you want time to do the things you want to do?

As you begin to do the things that will calm the chaos, you will take care of your responsibilities during the week and ask for help so you can reclaim your time. You will turn down invitations for happy hour on Friday night to lie in the tub and listen to music as you unwind from a busy week. You will invite a good friend out to lunch over the weekend with your newfound time. You will be more connected and healthy, achieving the things you need and want, loving your home, and experiencing more joy and ease than you have before.

Your behavior dictates your experiences. This is how alignment works.

Unfortunately, everyday life looks more like this...

You're living in complete chaos, working 50-hour weeks, with 10 hours commuting. Instead of going home when you're exhausted on Friday night, you go out for happy hour. You stay out too late and do some things you wish you hadn't. The next day, you wake up, do only what you need to do, then plop down in front of the television and knock out. When Monday comes, you know it's going to be more of the crappy same. You know you are never going to get where you said you wanted to go.

We say we want to calm the chaos, and we really do. But we don't do the things that will help us get what we want most. We do exactly the opposite, going for short-term payoffs rather than investing in long-term gains.

We are usually our own worst enemies in that we hurt ourselves by not doing the things we know we must do. We let other people and circumstances distract and influence us. We give away our power and leave our happiness in the control of others. We worry more about how people think of us than how we feel. None of these things serves our wellbeing.

Our bodies are designed to live 120 years, according to Dr. Walter M. Bortz, in his book, *We Live Too Short and Die Too Long*. However, because of the abuse our bodies sustain, we are not living as well or as long as we could. The stress of our success is literally killing us slowly by burying us with unrealized dreams and hopes.

Once you know what you want, you need to get into action and start doing what you say you want to do. If you want to learn a new skill, learn it. If you want to start a business, do it. Take the steps that will get you closer to what you say you want. Your desires come from an internal yearning. Give yourself permission to be inspired by them.

Behavior 5 | Be Disciplined

Discipline is a central behavior to achieve success at anything, at everything, in life. A Spiritual Girl must train her mind and character to build a sense of self-control and practice obedience.

Self-discipline is an articulation of freedom.

Being disciplined means doing what is necessary to do the things you say you are going to do, when you say you are going to do them, even when you don't feel like it. Those who feel consumed by the chaos and noise in the Material World lack clarity and, therefore, do not experience the freedom that comes with being disciplined to honor their dreams and deepest desires.

The more clarity you have about what you want and what it takes to help you achieve it, the easier it is to make supportive decisions. This means never thinking I wish, I could have, or I should have. This is the reason we will talk about and dig deep to discover what Living with Passion means to you and how to create it.

When you are disciplined, you activate your personal power to create more options and opportunities to live more freely. Discipline empowers you to invest your energy and talents to get what you want faster and easier than you thought possible. Whatever your desires, practicing discipline is essential to achieving them.

Behavior 6 | Be High Vibe

Have you ever been around someone who
is never happy or satisfied?

They complain about the most insignificant things, things you would never notice if they hadn't mentioned them. I swear it's a special power because, as the complainer complains, I lose all my mental capacity, eventually sitting unengaged, irritated, and unsure why.

When you Adopt a Thriving Mindset, you must use your mental strength to rise above negativity and see the insignificance of most things. I used to think we didn't have a choice in how to view the things that happened in our lives. They were either great or crappy. There was no in between.

If it was raining, it was a bad day.
If it was cold, it was a bad day.
If there was traffic, that sucked.
If there was housework to be done, that sucked.
If there were bills to pay, that sucked too.

But what I realize now that I didn't know then—and I think this goes for most of us—is we can choose to see these situations differently. We can choose to see them in a way that honors how we want to live and feel.

When you can choose high-vibe living, you stop letting things you cannot control, control you. You don't carry the heavy weight and emotional responsibility of everyone else's dramas. You work with purpose, knowing what you need and want to do, and do it all. You live passionately, open to the opportunities to enjoy more and laugh more, and you open the door to feeling more amazing things.

Just like anything else, it takes effort to do this because unexpected things happen. And they're not all going to be great. Ugly things will come into your experiences. Other people around you won't think the same way you do. People will talk about how they think you are, and not in a good way. They will talk about what they think you should do. They will talk about what you should have said. They talk—and that's all they do—because you are a reflection of what they desire but don't have the courage to create for themselves. Be the model for those who want to create a life worth living, but don't know what that means yet.

A situation may arise that no one has control of, such as an accident or the passing of a loved one. Yes, horrible things do happen, and that's when you most need to reaffirm your commitment to health, wealth, and happiness. Life happens. We cannot hide from it. We cannot think positive thoughts with the idea that they will protect us. We cannot always work our way around it. Sometimes, you have to go through some really tough drama and issues, and stop bandaging the problem. If you don't, it will leave you questioning the existence of a higher power and why you bother trying to be happy. When we don't deal with our drama and issues, this is what happens.

Our ability to choose how we want to feel in the face of all the chaos in the Material World makes the difference between something happening to you or something happening for you.

Choose to see the light.
Choose to find the lessons.
Choose to grow from all your experiences.
Choose not to let life happen in vain.

Don't let anything in this amazing life go to waste. Experience it all and remember to choose you, what you want, and how you want to live and feel. Choosing high-vibe living allows the love in you to grow from the inside out.

Today and every day, make a conscious decision to live from a good-feeling, high-vibe place. Do not give into the fear that brings on aggression, anger, resentment, or jealousy—all those lower vibe feelings and energy that do not allow you to feel good. They are fear dressed up as chaos.

Choose to feel good. When you do, you bring on feelings of pleasure, excitement, exhilaration, and enthusiasm—all those higher vibe feelings and energy we want to experience. These feelings are love dressed up as calm and synchronicity.

This doesn't mean you can never feel bad, because, guess what? We need to do that too. Sometimes we need to go through the mud to learn something. And when you do, you will come out better for it.

My only warning is don't park there. Give yourself permission to move through it. Let those emotions flow. Too often, we try to hold them, not let anyone see them. That's when they build up and cause the most damage and resistance. Give yourself permission to live in that place of fear and feel the things you need to feel, but do it with purpose. Get what you need to learn and move forward.

This isn't about being happy all the time or "acting" happy. We all have days when we have to give ourselves space to just be, low or high. Low-level energy days happen. We may feel crappy, moody, agitated. These feelings are the result of pushing too hard, not living in alignment, not letting go of past hurts, not creating more ease in our lives, and participating in the Material World's mini-melodramas that we create because of our fears and resistance. We can correct them and have fewer and fewer days when these things happen.

Love is a choice you make each day, in each moment. But when you don't feel it, don't do it. Gently get yourself there by giving yourself permission to honor your emotions. Then reach up for the next better emotion when you're ready.

Behavior 7 | Be Strategic

When we play games, we think strategically about how we can win. Although life is not a game, we still have to think strategically about how we can win each and every day, when making all our decisions—where to go, what to do, what to say and to whom, while simultaneously considering our true desires.

Start by asking yourself, "What is it I want to achieve," and "Will this get me closer to what I want?" Asking these questions will make it easier for you to determine if you are acting in your best interests.

Not having a strategy to live your life is like playing a game, but not playing to win. This is not about making moves that feel good right now. It's about making the best moves for your best life.

* * *

When you cultivate behaviors to Adopt a Thriving Mindset, you reclaim your personal power and open yourself to looking at the world from a different perspective. There is no more pretending you feel happy and well when you don't. You don't experience controlling, negative thoughts that cause bad feelings or bad behavior. Decisions are made with ease and in alignment with what will serve you and what you want to do.

To continue making progress in the areas of your life that you want to change, continue integrating the Principles of a Thriving Mindset. Practice being aware, willing, and committed each day.

SPIRITUAL PRESCRIPTION FOR COMMITMENT

The antidote for reconciling your behavior with who you want to be.

I am committed to creating a life worth living.

Many of us engage in our lives on a daily basis without giving much thought to how we want others to experience us. It is natural to want to be likable. To go somewhere and feel welcomed. I'd like to take this a step further, and with that in mind, ask:

How do you want to show up in the world?
Have you ever thought about it?
Did you know you had a choice?

This is about how you want to engage with the Material World, how you want people to think of and experience you. You want to be your authentic self, but who is that? That's what you're here to define for yourself. Clarity in life gives you the ability to focus on what matters.

Reflection | Find Your Words

Thinking about your higher self, how do you want other people to describe you? Knowing this will help you respond, react, and take actions that honor how you want to be remembered.

What three words describe the best of who you want to be?

Word 1:

Why did you choose this word?
Why is this word important to you?

Word 2:

Why did you choose this word?

Why is this word important to you?

Word 3:

Why did you choose this word?
Why is this word important to you?

Use these words to guide your thoughts, actions, and interactions each day. When necessary, reconcile your behavior with how you want to be remembered.

Once you have your words, prepare a loving daily reminder to keep you aligned with how you want to be felt during interactions and remembered afterwards.

Chapter 5

Live with Purpose

"Most of us spend too much time on what is urgent
and not enough time on what is important."
~Stephen R. Covey

If you have practiced the Spiritual Prescriptions presented so far, your mindset and your thinking should be coming into alignment with the way you want to live. This may take some repetition, some rereading, and a lot of patience. After all, this isn't easy work. But it is meaningful and life-changing work.

As you learned in Chapter 4, Living with Passion allows you to see things differently. When things don't feel good, connect with your passion, and choose to see your experience with eyes of love, fully connected to that person you truly are.

Now that you have committed to Living with Passion with a Thriving Mindset, you are ready to take on the second critical component of the Flight Plan: Live with Purpose. To do this, we must calm the CHAOS and fully focus on the parts of life that make it more fulfilling and worthwhile.

Calm the CHAOS

The CHAOS in the Material World blocks our inner Spiritual Girl from connecting with what she desires. In this chapter, you will begin to calm that CHAOS. You will discover how to Live with Purpose, as discovered and defined by you. I'm not going to tell you what to do in order to live with purpose. Rather, you will define your purpose through your own exploration of what it will take to create YOUR life worth living. By doing so, you will begin to make a positive impact on the quality of your health, wealth, and happiness by removing the barriers that keep you from achieving what is possible.

Based on studies in wellbeing about things such as what improves our longevity and quality of life, I have pinpointed 5 elements to help us calm the CHAOS and achieve work-life balance in this Material World so we can Live with Purpose. By purpose, I mean focused each day on the things that increase your health, wealth, and happiness. These are not separate. They all contribute to the same emotional compass. They are:

Connection
Health and Wellness
Achievement
Organization
Spirituality

For too long, our society has accepted that work-life balance is some big myth, something no one can actually achieve. I want you to know that's all a load of crap, pure and simple. Stop buying into the notion that you cannot have or achieve work-life balance!

You see, work-life balance is not about equality; it's about equity. While we may crave the same things, we crave them in different amounts. As humans in a collective experience, we share the same chemistry and physiology, but we are unique in our expression and experience. Anyone who tells you that you cannot achieve work-life balance doesn't see you or the big picture.

We deal with tons of guilt, worry, and neglect. What we have to look at is why.

Why are you feeling guilty about missing something or not doing enough? Why are you worried about losing your job or your business? Why are you neglecting the people who mean the most to you, including yourself?

Since The Illness, I've learned a lot about living a balanced life. Does this mean I've mastered it and never screw up? No, it doesn't. I'm not perfect; I'm human just like you. But what this does mean for me is I quickly notice when I get knocked out, so I can fix it right away and return to my center.

Stop accepting surviving as the default for living a life well-lived, because you deserve more.

The Five Elements of Living with Purpose

Following are the Five Elements of Living with Purpose that help you calm the chaos in the Material World.

Element 1 | Connection – Creating and having strong relationships and love in your life.

Connection begins with you—how well you connect to what you like and want for yourself, and how well you connect to your family, your friends, and the community, the Material World.

Element 2 | Health and Wellness – Having good mental and physical health and enough energy to get things done on a daily basis.

Health and wellness mean taking good care of your mental and physical environments by nourishing them when they need nourishment. When you drink water, eat regularly, and create healthy boundaries, you can engage your health and wellness at a whole new level of performance and accuracy.

Element 3 | Achievement – Investing your time and liking what you do every day.

Achievement means striving to improve and create new, higher standards of excellence for yourself. It means being a lifelong learner. Our desire for achievement is what drives us to discover our full potential.

Element 4 | Organization – Effectively managing your life.

Organization means having a place for everything and having everything in its place. It is not about being clean and tidy. It's about having what you need where you need it.

Element 5 | Spirituality – Engaging enthusiastically with your daily experiences.

When I speak about spirituality, I mean a sense of connection to something bigger than yourself, which involves a search for meaning.

There comes a time—mine came when I was thirty-eight, and I thought I was dying—when we ask ourselves, "Is this all there is?" Spirituality helps us cope a devastating reality so we can be happy with the answers to the questions we ask ourselves when we feel like our end of time is near. Questions like, "Did I matter to anyone other than myself? Did I love fully and openly? Did I truly live to my potential?"

Each day, engage in the five elements to Calm the CHAOS, in the amount of time that feels good to you to maintain a feeling of calm and focus. Most of us want this. REALLY. Want. This. And never get it. Unfortunately, it's because most refuse to take responsibility for their happiness. They believe happiness is something they get, not something they create. They believe someone can give them the secret ingredient to create wellbeing in their lives.

They are distracted.
They are distracted by their cell phones.
They are distracted by their obligations and responsibilities.
They are distracted by their unsatisfied needs.

When someone tells me everything is fine in their world in one breath and in the next, they share the chaos in their life and then end with the fact that they are okay surviving from day to day, I just about crawl out of my skin.

Are you kidding me? Okay? Okay is not great. Okay is not good. It's that survivor mindset that tells you it is.

We must calm the C H A O S to quiet the noise of our Material World to find a path that feels good.

If we hope to thrive, we must find ways to overcome our challenges, to get those golden nuggets of wisdom, and to put them to good use. That's the only way to ensure we don't repeat those cycles of life we don't enjoy. The five Elements to Living with Purpose will guide you and help you identify what matters as you define what a life worth living means to you.

If we take intentional action in these five areas, we will quiet the noise and get on a path that feels good. Each element plays its part in achieving and maintaining your wellbeing.

Our emotions act as guideposts. When we feel good, we are on the right path. When we don't, we're not. If you ignore those feelings, you expose yourself and your body to dis-ease. Although we are composed of the same matter, we have genetics, history, and beliefs that make us unique. So, while all five elements must be present in our lives, we crave them in varying amounts.

If you integrate the five elements into your lifestyle each day in the levels you desire, you will be happier and more satisfied. You will achieve and maintain your wellbeing, allowing you to respond with grace to the fires burning all around you. Those fires will always burn, but you will not be charred or consumed by them.

Moving Forward – Monique

Monique is an accountant. She was one of the first people to put The Flight Plan to work in her life. When she came to me, she hated her work job. She was frustrated with the number of hours she worked and with the quality of her engagement at home and her relationship with her spouse. She was contemplating walking away from everything, calling it quits on her career, her marriage, and her life.

Together, we examined what was going on for her. From my sessions with Monique, I could see she had no boundaries or structure. She loved her husband and their life but didn't love the loneliness and disconnection she felt. She worked so much she found no time to rest. It was no surprise to me to learn that she had high blood pressure, was fifty pounds overweight, and had recently learned she acquired diabetes.

Through working her Flight Plan, she discovered that she loved her work but wanted to scale back. She created a plan to develop a digital course teaching small business owners how to stay out of trouble with the IRS and best accounting practices. She also took her health more seriously, started eating better, and exercising too. After six months, she no longer suffered from high blood pressure, had released her extra weight, and no longer has diabetes.

* * *

A Spiritual Girl asks as lot of herself to create balance in her life. I wish I could tell you it is easy, but it isn't. If it were, we wouldn't have so much dis-ease in the Material World. I've done the work to get there and helped thousands of others do the same. I know it is well worth it, and you will too.

Now is the time to release the belief that you don't have a choice, because I am going to walk you through how to do it. One. Step. At. A. Time.

SPIRITUAL PRESCRIPTION FOR DIRECTION

Antidote for lack of direction to discover what you truly desire from life and for feeling completely lost and disconnected.

What I think matters. What I want matters. I matter.

Solidify your commitment to design your life consciously. It is important to understand any resistance or fears you have around making lifestyle changes to improve your engagement, enthusiasm, and excitement. It takes courage to stop accepting what you receive by default.

All types of opportunities will present themselves, but it is up to you to select which are right for the life you are consciously and deliberately designing. Don't let taking the easy route for short-term gains keep you from experiencing greater joy by going the distance for what you really want.

Both deficiency and abundance exist in our lives. This is a call to stop focusing on the beliefs that leave you powerless to change your path. Remember, this is not about taking just ANY path, but, instead, about getting on THE path to Passion, Purpose, and Play.

When we feel unhappy, at best we make changes in our environment. We move, change our work, or leave our significant others before we take a good look within ourselves. Once we conquer our beliefs, thoughts, and behaviors that no longer serve us, we find that transformation for the better in our environment happens without much effort.

Reflection | Where Are You Now

Your emotions are guideposts along the path from where you are to where you want to be.

Three times a day, each day, ask yourself,

> **On a scale from 1 to 10 (1 being not well and 10 being elated), how do I feel right now?**

Then dig deeper. Ask yourself:

> **Why am I feeling this way?**
> **Where do I feel this in my body?**
> **What can I do to raise that number?**

It's important to know where you are by being present in your experiences so you can gauge your feelings to determine if that is where you want to be. If we want to raise our numbers, we must look for a more loving view. This keeps us from getting sucked into the distraction and disconnection that keeps us from realizing what we desire most. This is not about changing your external environment as much as it is about changing your internal environment by holding a more loving perspective.

Calm the CHAOS ~ Connection

> *"In everyone's life, at some time, our inner fire goes out.*
> *Then it bursts into flames by an encounter with another*
> *human being. We should all be thankful for those people*
> *who rekindle the Inner Spirit." ~Albert Schweitzer*

The first Element of Living with Purpose is Connection. As a society, many of us spend more time picking our soap than we spend selecting the people in whom we invest time. Like most things in our lives, we allow connections to happen by default, even when our resulting relationships don't make us feel good.

Brene Brown, in her book ***Gifts of Imperfection***, defines connection perfectly as "The energy that exists between people when they feel seen, heard, and valued; when they can give, and receive without judgment; and when they derive sustenance and strength from the relationship."

Because we feed off the energy of those around us, we must consider those we surround ourselves with and understand…

> **Who are the people with whom I want to**
> **devote my time and attention?**
> **How much time do I want to invest in my relationships?**

We all want to feel connected to those who surround us. With many thanks to social media, we have more opportunity for connection than we ever have, yet the numbers on those who feel alone continue to rise.

> With how many of those virtual connections
> would you share your day's high or low?

Until just over a decade ago, our friends consisted of people in our immediate space—where we worked, where we lived, and where we played. Finding real friends was much easier; we usually had only a handful of people to consider.

Nothing influences your levels of happiness
as much as your relationships with your spouse and significant others.

To achieve connection, we give some people more time than they deserve. We compromise how we want to feel by keeping negative, energy-draining, soul-sucking friends we should have dropped long ago. We must be careful with these types of connections. They can disconnect us from how we want to feel and what we want for ourselves.

The results of a survey published in 2010 by the AARP (American Association of Retired Persons) indicated that more than one in three Americans over age 45 identifies as being chronically lonely.

We all want to feel seen, heard, and valued, and when we don't, we feel rejected, separate from everyone and everything.

When we connect, our bodies send signals to our brains and initiate releases of "feel" good hormones: dopamine, vasopressin, oxytocin; and we feel euphoric.

I don't know about you, but I love the natural buzz I get when I allow
life to light me up.

Many people don't understand how their connections affect their overall wellbeing. Study after study is finding that the quality of our immediate connections is one of the most important factors in our overall satisfaction with life.

A 2010 study called the "Social Relationship and Mortality Risk" revealed that friendships have as much impact on the risk of death as smoking, drinking, or obesity. Other studies have shown that people with at least five intimate relationships, those they can share their personal stories with without fear of judgment, are happier and live longer than those who do not. The better the quality of our friendships, the more ambition, growth, and stability we experience in our lives.

According to Gallup News Service, the average American in 2004 had nine close friends. A 2010 study by Assistant Professor of Sociology Matthew Brashears of Cornell University shows 29% have more than two, 18% have two, 48% have one, and 4% have no intimate relationships.

The average American has one or two close connections.

When I was sick, I felt forgotten. The Illness was incredibly isolating and lonely. For a couple of months, people called out of concern. As things lingered, the calls stopped. Family and friends quit coming by and checking in. I longed for someone who could or wanted to understand. I couldn't put any more on my husband's shoulders. He was alone, doing the best he could. I could see my children struggling, and I was helpless. No one stepped in to help us. This brought me clarity about the connections I wanted to create and foster in my life.

I want supportive, close, deep friendships; I will settle for nothing else. Another gift of The Illness was seeing the value of my relationships and their impact on my wellbeing. This forced me to renegotiate the expectations from my relationships. Some healed, others did not. Several would never recover and, to this day, have not been mended.

These were realities I took responsibility for creating in my life. Yet, that's not where I started. For about a year, I was bitter and angry because I didn't understand why I had created shallow relationships with those I loved and in whom I invested time. Was my family that easily forgotten about? Was I?

Sources of Connection

There are two sources of connection. Family and intimate relationships are the primary source of meaningful connections, and friendships are a secondary source.

Family and Intimate Relationships, and Friendships

Family are those we were raised by and with, and those who have a strong influence in our lives.

Intimate relationships, or close relationships, are those we rely on to get through our days. They are the people we trust and call on when we want to celebrate or need support.

Friendships are those who are present in our lives, but we don't necessarily rely on these relationships to get through the day.

It is easy and natural to want our relationships to mean as much to the other party as they mean to us. We want them to care about and respect us as much as we care about and respect them. But relationships are rarely equal. This is an expectation we must release. Relationships are not tit-for-tat. We must not keep score.

We must allow our connections to show up as who they are, which can mean they won't always show up the way we need them to, if at all. If we want them in our lives, we must accept them for who they are and seek to create the type of relationship that will serve and not hurt us. This takes knowing what you need and want from the people in your life and creating boundaries. While this may seem like an act of selfishness, it is actually an act of self-love.

Some friendships can become incredibly intimate, while relationships with some family members can be similar to friendships, or even less familiar and attached. Know where you want to fit people into your life. This has more to do with how you feel about the people in your life than about the status of your blood relation. As your life fills, invest your time in connections that make a positive impact on your wellbeing.

Deepen Connections

Create the time it takes to build the ties that bind. Don't be one of those friends who says, "Let's get together!" then never does. Don't say things you don't mean. If this is important to you, if they are important to you, you should create time to foster, nurture, and deepen your connections.

> How long has it been since you had a quiet
> dinner with someone you love . . .
> When was the last time you had a heart-to-
> heart with one of your children . . .
> . . . not because something was wrong, but
> because you wanted to connect?

My life, like the lives of my friends and clients, has been filled with missed opportunities to bond more closely with my spouse, children, family, and friends. We all want to connect, but somehow it doesn't happen. Thus, the weakest of your relationships can fall apart easily.

For me, once infrequent calls and dinners became non-existent. Evenings were no longer filled with laughter around the kitchen table or watching a movie with my husband and children. I was so wrapped up in what was going on in my world, it kept me from seeing what was going on in their world.

If I knew then what I know now, that would have been the first clue I was lost in the chaos. When you are connected, you don't have separate worlds. Feeling separate is a huge sign that you are disconnected.

It makes complete sense that the more someone disconnects and pulls away from their relationships, the more isolated they feel, giving them the exact opposite of what they need and want. Yet, that's what many do.

I can wholeheartedly say, because of this recognition, I have a new appreciation for my time and the quality of my relationships. I focus on those who fill me with joy with no apology, and I implore you to do the same.

When you feel separate and disconnected, honor those feelings. Take the time you need and give people the time they require. We all need quiet time to process, and it's okay to ask for this time without fear of judgment.

There are two ways to deepen the connections you have with the people in your life. The first way is by accident, chance, or tragedy. The second is by design. It is essential to do the work of defining what you want from your connections or relationships.

Make it a priority to keep in touch with the people you love. Don't be one of those friends who says, "We should get together more often," as you keep moving. If you don't mean it, don't say it. Be the friend who says, "Let's go out for dinner," and then makes plans to do so. It's okay to say, "It's so good to see you," and leave it at that. Honesty is how you create strong ties. Drop the BS. You owe it to yourself and your connections to be honest.

Design Your Connections

You alone can determine and define what YOU want in your life from your connections. Here are a few ideas to deepen the connections that make life worth living.

Create Play Time Rituals

Do something regularly that bonds you with your connections. Plan a recurring coffee, lunch, or dinner. Make it more fun by adding something everyone enjoys or finds relaxing, such as a massage or going for a walk. Plan something out of the ordinary such as skydiving or a cooking class. The point is to do something together, often.

Check In

Get in touch more frequently with those you want to deepen connections with. Start by sharing how much you appreciate them. Share something exciting or fun that happened that day or week. You can make these meetings daily, a couple times a week, weekly, or as often as you want. Do what feels good for you.

Keep in Touch

Make an effort to keep in touch with new and old friends alike. Use Facebook, Twitter, or other social media networks to keep in touch. However, make it a point also to reach out personally from time to time to keep your relationships meaningful and fulfilling.

Give 'Em a Break

I know this seems obvious, but it must be said, because if you care about someone, you listen. Give them the benefit of the doubt if trouble ensues. Do not take things your friends do personally. Don't get upset if a friend is late, cancels plans at the last minute, or forgets about something important to you. Perhaps your friend is just overwhelmed and being a friend means giving them the benefit of the doubt.

Say What You Mean and Mean What You Say

Too often, we hold back. We hold back how much we love our friends. We hold back how much we appreciate their companionship. We hold back our hurt feelings. Keep the lines of communication open and honest to keep your ties strong and significant.

Be Nice

Talk to the people you care about. Be interested in their lives. Be nice to them. Be kind. Reach out and see how they are doing. If things go awry, don't talk about them; talk to them. It happens, and when it does, don't let things build up until you cannot communicate clearly and from a place of love. The key is to be someone you enjoy spending time with, and people will want to devote more time to you.

When good things happen to your friends, be excited for them. Let them celebrate and support them enthusiastically. Always look for the positive, share big belly laughs, and give authentic praise. We all want to be appreciated, heard, and seen.

Show Up

If you want meaningful friendships, make time to see your friends in person. We are all busy, so don't use your busyness as an excuse. If it's important to you, create time in your schedule to visit with a friend at least once a month for dinner, lunch, or a visit to the local farmers' market. Make it stress-free and fun.

Put It Away

Turn off your cell phone and digital devices. Get rid of anything that keeps you connected to anywhere else other than where you are. This prevents you from enjoying the company of a real live person. Not doing so will squash any chance of a meaningful relationship and raise your stress meter.

A 2012 two-year study of technology use and moods of 1,367 women and men at the University of Wisconsin-Milwaukee found those who sent and received the most calls and messages were also most likely to say this connection left them tired and distracted at home.

In your personalized Flight Plan, CREATE time for investing in your connections. I have an alarm that goes off every Wednesday at 10 a.m., asking me, "Who are you going to connect with?" This reminds me how important my relationships are and to make that call and plan for that coffee or dinner. Otherwise, like everyone else, I get distracted and let too much time go by. Would something like this work for you? Try it. Set an alarm now. Be intentional and create a chance to cultivate meaningful connections.

When They Don't Support You

Unfortunately, not everyone is where you are, and it can be challenging to be around others who are not. We all have a family member or friend, or several, who just can't help themselves. You know, the person who does things that don't make sense and are kind of hurtful but fail to see it.

This is what it may look like:

> ***A friend who doesn't value you.*** She seems to treat everyone respectfully and kindly, except you. She's not quite as kind to you, as if your friendship is not as important as others or as if you don't measure up.

> ***A friend who compares and competes with you.*** When something good happens for you, something better has happened for her, always. When something bad happens for you, something worse happens to her. It's always a competition, good or bad.

> ***A friend who is brutally honest.*** She tells you as it is, but her words are harsh and judgmental. They don't feel like they come from a good, loving place.

> ***A friend who is always negative.*** The cup is always half empty for her. She complains about everything and everyone, even when she volunteers and is doing good things. Nothing's good enough. She is not happy, and she makes everyone around her unhappy too.

> ***A friend who uses you.*** She knows you have amazing people and friends in your life and is always asking you to reach out on her behalf. In and of itself, this is not a problem.

However, that's the only time you hear from her, when she needs something from you, and she never asks how things are going in your world.

Each of these situations can make you want to be done with this person and relationship. No one would blame you. There are many ways we get hurt in relationships. There are also lots of ways our friendships nurture us, and that's why they are worth the effort.

We must acknowledge how difficult it is for people with different experiences, cultures, and influences to come together. We all have lovable and not so lovable parts of our being. Those "not so lovable" parts are the shadow sides of our character. We all have them. Some you will want to work on; others you won't. These are not part of who we are. They are habits. And just like any other habit, you can modify them so they are more pleasing to you, or you can completely get rid of them.

If people tell you that an aspect of your character is an issue, you may decide you like it and keep it. People can then decide for themselves if they like being with you, given those qualities. That's the way it works. I'm not saying you have to change to be more likable, but you do have to decide what you want for yourself.

Be Selfish

When you are in a situation with a family member or a friend, ask yourself,

"What is the value of this relationship?"

The answer to this question is paramount. When I have asked myself this, I have crossed off very few people. But I have drifted from lots of people for many reasons, some of those I stated above and worse.

At the end of the day, we need connections, and our relationships with family and friends are essential to our wellbeing. Know that doesn't mean you have to let someone treat you poorly.

Decide what you want to do about this relationship. This is your life, and you have to determine who is worth investing time and energy with and who isn't.

Do you love this person and not see life without them?

Do you enjoy your time with this person and think they really have no idea how hurtful they can be?

Do you have a lot of common friends and need to find a way to be peaceful for their sake?

Think about it. Let these questions guide your actions.

There are dozens of reasons we keep difficult people around. Believe me, I have my fair share, and I'm sure I'm one of those people for someone else. We all are. It's the cycle of life. Stick with those who make you feel good. Anything that doesn't feel right isn't.

The power of good friendships increases your health, wealth, and happiness. However, all relationships are not equal. Know who you want in your life now. Let them come and go without expectation or judgment.

Create a Peace Posse

A Peace Posse is a group of people you choose to share your life with. These qualify as your intimate relationships.

10 Roles for Your Peace Posse

Things happen; when they do, where, or more importantly, who do you turn to?

You may be wondering what types of friendships we need or what roles we need our friends to fill in our lives. This is where your Peace Posse comes in.

Role 1 | The Work Friend. This friend is essential to making it in your work environment. This friend is good for your productivity and helps your day go faster.

Role 2 | The Dependable Friend. This friend's loyalty knows no bounds; they will go to the ends of the earth for you, and you would do the same for them.

Role 3 | The Know-It-All Friend. If you belong to a group and aren't as involved as you would like to be, this friend has you covered. She keeps you in touch and tells you about special events, so you never feel left out.

Role 4 | The Forever Friend. No judgment, no excuses. This friend knows and loves all of you—the good, the bad, and the ugly (including where the bodies are buried), and would never betray your trust.

Role 5 | The Let's Do It Friend. When you want to check out a new restaurant or a new movie, this is the friend you call. You share the same interests and sensibilities.

Role 6 | The Stay-In Friend. This friend is happy to do nothing with you. This is the person you call when you want to hang out. No entertainment needed, your company is enough.

Role 7 | The Life Coach Friend. You go to this friend when you need an ear and some loving encouragement. They help you sort out an issue or just listen to you vent and give you the courage to go after what you want.

Role 8 | The Tough Friend. This boldly honest friend will tell you exactly as it is and with love. From the man you're with, to the color of your skirt, she gives it to you straight so you can be your best.

Role 9 | The Disconnected Friend. She has no kids to worry about, she's not attached, and when you need to escape, she's there. She won't ask why you need that third four-olive nasty dirty martini.

Role 10 | The Good Times (Only) Friend. When you want to go out for drinks and guarantee you'll have a great time and lots of big belly laughs, you call this friend. Easy, breezy, just how you need it—when you need it.

You may have more than one friend in multiple roles, and you may have some roles that are open at this time. As you may have noticed, making friends as an adult is not as easy as when you were ten, but that doesn't mean you shouldn't try to create your Peace Posse.

Move Forward with Challenging Connections

We will want to continue some connections in our lives for our own reasons, even when they are challenging. Perhaps it's a sibling, a parent, or a longtime friend you are not ready to give up on. Here are a few ideas for how to move forward with those connections.

Try again. Things happen, and when they do, we need to be able to put them aside, especially if the transgression was small and incidental. If a friend shows up a little late for lunch or if they don't return your call, don't take it personally. Ask them what is going on. If what happened isn't really a big deal, just let it go. Move forward.

Renegotiate. Some people will step all over your boundaries. They push you and demand more and more resources from you. You know the type; they are needy and just don't see it. Have a sit-down. Tell them how you feel about your friendship and what you need from them.

I have found having these sit-downs honors my worthiness, which is entirely the opposite of what relationships like this make you feel. Be forewarned, there are times when I have had these conversations then moved on to the next step below. When you can't come to a mutual understanding, that's when you know it's time.

Let go. When relationships are just not salvageable for one reason or another, it's okay to let them go. When you do, let go with love. There doesn't have to be anger and resentment. There can be a common understanding that the two of you should not be very involved, if at all.

Forgiveness

It's important to understand forgiveness so you can move forward, especially when a connection is more than difficult and hurts you. How to forgive and let go is not as simple as it seems, but getting caught up in the blame and pain is a trap.

Feelings of anger and resentment do not feel good. Everything gets heavier. The sun doesn't shine as brightly. Our food loses its flavor. Everything we do seems to come out a hot mess.

I used to see posts on Facebook or Twitter saying, "Just let go and forgive." I'd think to myself, "Yeah right. That sounds great but HOW do you do that?" Before The Illness, I gave forgiveness very little thought. Until then, I didn't know what forgiveness meant. It's a magnificent idea to let go and forgive. IF. YOU. CAN.

I wanted to know exactly how to forgive someone genuinely and how that could make someone feel better and happier. I so deeply wanted to feel better inside and let go of decades of hurt I had carried on my back like treasure in a deep-sea shipwreck. Carrying it wasn't helping me feel healthy, wealthy, or happy. It was keeping me from creating a life worth living.

In discussions with clients and friends, I realized everyone doesn't have the same understanding about what forgiveness is and isn't. Simply put, *forgiveness is a grant of pardon and ceasing to feel resentment against a person.* Many withhold forgiveness because they don't want to let the other person off the hook. However, forgiveness has nothing to do with the person you are forgiving. When you understand what forgiveness truly is, you can release the pain and forgive more freely.

Forgiveness is not acting as if nothing has happened. Something did happen. Understand the lesson that caused the hurt, so it's not repeated.

Forgiveness is not excusing the person for their actions. We only excuse someone when they are not to blame for a wrong-doing.

Forgiveness is not letting someone continue to hurt you. Demand that the company you keep treat you well and respect your boundaries.

Forgiveness is not condoning harmful behavior yesterday, today, or tomorrow. It is never acceptable for someone to treat you as if you are not valuable.

Forgiveness is not reconciling. Whether or not you allow someone back into your life that you have forgiven is entirely up to you.

Once I realized what forgiveness was NOT, moving forward and letting go became so much easier. There was so much to forgive and let go. In my life, I became a pro at holding on to hurt. It took me over two years to reconcile with those from whom I had withheld forgiveness.

Now that we know what forgiveness isn't, let's look at how we can forgive.

How to Forgive

First, you must ***acknowledge*** why you are hurt and allow the feelings that come up because of it to arise. No matter what the situation, how you feel is valid. Don't ignore how you feel.

Second, communicate with love. When you are ready, express the pain you feel to the person who hurt you without yelling or attacking. Don't shout, throw things, hit, or bring things up that you have already moved beyond. Moving forward is harder when you drag all your old baggage with you.

Third, get clarity about the situation and attempt to ***understand*** how and why the situation that hurt you unfolded. Was there a misunderstanding or was the hurt intentional? Understanding what happened not only brings closure, but it allows you to truly receive the benefit of knowing, not assuming, what was thought, felt, or said. Realize, our assumptions normally have no basis in fact.

Fourth, *protect* yourself from being hurt again. Before you forgive, you need to know that you will not be a victim again. What will make you feel safe moving forward? Do new boundaries need to be established? Do you need an apology, reassurance, or distance? Whatever it is, ask for it. Don't assume the other person will know what you need.

Fifth, take responsibility and *forgive* yourself for your role. As they say, "It takes two to tango." Accept responsibility for any part you may have had in the situation that you want to forgive, and forgive yourself for it too. Assuming responsibility for the condition of your life is essential. Think of what you could have done differently to avoid the situation and what you can do if this situation comes up again with the same person or someone else.

Sixth, **decide** how to handle the relationship moving forward. This is where you get to be completely selfish and decide what you want from this relationship. Do you want to reconcile and hope things will go back to the way they were, or do you need a new normal? Another option is ending the relationship altogether. Do what you feel is best for you and the way you want to live.

Last, *let go* and overtly forgive, verbally or in writing. Speaking or writing out the words "I forgive you" is incredibly healing.

Forgiveness is truly the gift we give ourselves.

By releasing the pain and resentment, we make a promise to ourselves to move forward, and when we do, we feel better. Holding on to grudges or clinging to betrayals and disappointments is bad for our minds, bodies, and souls.

According to a 2005 study in the *Journal of Behavioral Medicine*, forgiving those who have wronged us lowers blood pressure, cholesterol, and heart rate. It also reduces levels of depression, anxiety, and anger.

Kind of cool, right? This is the way it works.
As you do things to make yourself better emotionally, you feel better mentally and physically.

Communication

Do you ever watch people argue and think, if only they would listen to each other, all their issues would be resolved?

I have listened to stories of siblings, spouses, and friends miscommunicating. Standing on the outside looking in, it's always easy to see how the fire was ignited. However, when you're mixed up in the situation, you can't see what's on the tip of your nose.

The discipline of communication focuses on how we use messages to generate meaning within and across various contexts, cultures, channels, and media. It's the act of transferring information. This can be vocal (using your voice); written (books, magazines, websites, or emails); visual (logos, images, maps, charts, or graphs); or non-verbal (body language, gestures, and the tone and pitch of your voice).

How well this information is transmitted and received is a measure of how effective our communication skills are.

Communication skills affect all aspects of your life, from your professional to your social life and everything between. The ability to communicate accurately, clearly, and as intended is a vital life skill and something that is often overlooked. It's never too late to work on your communication skills, and doing so can improve the quality and understanding of your relationships.

Every healthy relationship includes open, honest communication. Following are a few ways to open the channels of communication in your relationships. Please use caution when applying these ideas. You know your relationships best, and if any of these would put your relationship in danger, don't use them.

Healthy relationships deserve the benefit of the doubt. Open communication, no matter the situation, is essential in creating strong ties. This is how you keep the peace. This is how you keep the joy. This is how you keep the love.

The Right Time

If you have an issue you want to discuss and are ready for a serious conversation, pick the right time to start the conversation. I ask the person I want to speak to when would be a good time for them to sit and talk. Do not start meaningful conversations by walking into a room and demanding to speak now or by yelling. It won't go well.

Face-to-Face

Avoid talking about serious issues or matters in writing. Text messages, letters, and emails can be misinterpreted. Speak in person so that unnecessary miscommunications do not inflame the situation. Having said that, some people are more comfortable writing their thoughts; if that's the case for you, go ahead and write your thoughts out. Reading your letter aloud to the other person is a good way to start the conversation when you don't know how to start.

No Attacking

Choose a way to share, with love, what you are feeling. Beginning the conversation with words like "you" sounds like you are in attack mode and will make the other person defensive. If they get defensive, they are less likely to be receptive to your message. Instead, use, "I feel." As an example, instead of saying, "You never listen," say, "I feel you never listen." It does make a difference in how your message is delivered and received.

Be Honest

Sometimes, the truth hurts. But that is no reason not to share it. Being able to share your truth in your relationships is essential to its wellness. There is nothing you can't say in a loving way. You don't ever need to be brutal. If you have made a mistake, and it is possible—no one is perfect—take responsibility and apologize, instead of making excuses.

Check Your Body

When you speak, make eye contact. Sit up and face the person you are talking to. Let the other person know you are listening. Show them you really care about how they feel. Listen and respond.

The Two-Day Rule

If someone does something to hurt or anger you, you need to talk about it, but you don't have to have that conversation right away. If you're still upset after two days, say something. If not, consider letting it go. Remember, no one can read your mind. If you don't talk when you're upset, there's no way for them to know what they did. Once you share your feelings and the other person apologizes, or you come to a resolution, let it go, which means not bringing up resolved issues when they are no longer relevant.

Now, sometimes things really anger you, and that's okay. It happens. Here's how to go about communicating when it's time to confront the hurt.

Stop. Take a step back and breathe. Give yourself time to calm down. Sometimes taking a break from a situation can keep it from getting worse.

Think. Reflect on the situation and what triggered you. Figure out the real issue and think of a way to explain your feelings.

Talk. When you're ready . . . have a conversation using what I shared in the points above.

Listen. After you share your feelings, stop talking and listen to what the other person has to say. You both deserve the opportunity to express your feelings and points of view.

Communicating is not always easy. Some of what I share here may feel awkward when you first try, but these tips will help you improve your communication and build healthier relationships.

Be Authentic

Do you ever feel like someone you have known for
ages doesn't like or understand you anymore?

When you take the time to grow, you expect excellent things to come from that, right? Good things do come, but no longer being on the same page with those you hang out with can make you feel angry, resentful, or guilty.

Give yourself a break. Relationships come and go, especially when people grow, change jobs, move from one neighborhood to another, or die. I don't mean to be morbid, but all relationships have a beginning, a middle, and an end. We must get comfortable with that.

This doesn't mean you have to cut ties or be nasty to anyone. You can move on peacefully and with love.

Here are **Three Things to Ask Before You Leave Someone Behind.**

Is this natural? There is a time and place for everything and everyone. Naturally, when you take on new things, you will evolve. Isn't that the point? And when you do, you may realize you no longer have much in common with the friends you hang with. Change is growth, and growth is good.

Is this really the end? Meet people where they are. Just as you are on a path, so is the person you are in a relationship with. Your journeys may continue in different directions, and that's okay. You never know, your paths may cross again.

Am I being a snob? Always be the model, a shining example of who you aspire to surround yourself with. Learning, growing, and having new experiences is part of the process of living. However, we each do it in our own way. As you seek out personal growth in your life, don't become a snob and judge others for not doing the same or agreeing with you. If we all did things the same way at the same time, life would be less interesting, wouldn't it? Embrace the uniqueness that makes us all special.

As you adopt a more evolved version of yourself, treat others with the compassion, love, and understanding you desire.

Moving on doesn't have to be hard. It's as simple as finding other things to fill your time. You can still catch up with missed friends when the timing is right. As our lives and priorities change, our friends will too. It's okay.

* * *

When it comes to connections, one of the most important things to remember is not getting caught up in the drama. You can only control yourself. Fulfill yourself by spending time with those who mean the most to you, those you want to reconnect with, and those you want to surround yourself with. These people will change throughout your life and when they do, honor them. Don't hold judgment or hurt feelings. Everyone has their own path, and as you embrace your path, others will embrace theirs. Move on with love.

In this section, I have asked you to examine the connections you have and the quality of those connections. As you gain clarity about who you want to be, how you want to feel, and what you want, the relationships that support you will become evident. This will allow you to purposely focus your energy on connections that matter to you most.

SPIRITUAL PRESCRIPTION FOR MEANINGFUL CONNECTIONS

Antidote for feeling misunderstood and unsupported in your relationships.

I desire and am deserving of meaningful connections and deep relationships.

Are you fulfilled by your connections?

Every day is a gift; unfortunately, it is a limited gift, lasting only 24 hours. That time must be invested effectively to connect with those who make a positive impact on your health, wealth, and happiness.

Now that you know the kinds of connections that make a positive impact on your wellbeing, it is time to get clear about your relationships and how you feel about them. Take an inventory of the relationships you value.

What do you want to experience from and with your family and friends? How do you want to show up in interactions with them? What kind of impact do you want to have in their lives?

Reflection | Create an Inventory

Write the names of your family and friends on a sheet of paper. I know this seems tedious, but an inventory of your relationships will support you in creating a fulfilled and meaningful life. I've said it before, and I am sure I will say it again: This is work. But, oh, . . . it is so worth it.

Next, from the list of family and friends, consider:

How many close relationships do I have?
How often do I see the people who matter to me?
How often do we speak?

Then, rate your family and friends based on how you feel when you are around them; use a scale from 1 to 5, with 1 being low or draining and 5 being inspired or joyous.

For those who did not rate a 5, answer the following:

How well does this person know me?
How supportive is this person?
Do they encourage me to be a better person?
How much does this relationship mean to me?
Do I want to invest more time and
energy into this relationship?

Read through your thoughts.

Are you satisfied with the numbers?
Do the numbers show you are feeling
supported, understood, and connected?
What did you discover about your immediate circle of friends?

Please understand that I am not suggesting you "break up" with your family and friends. There will be relationships you value and don't want to release despite their rating. When it comes to those relationships, set boundaries that will help you maintain a relationship that will not place you at risk for sacrificing your wellbeing. You can gradually allow distance to grow between you and those individuals who you have determined are not good for you and do not support you in the ways you want to be supported.

My relationship with my father is complex. Michael has hurt me several times and in so many ways; however, this is a relationship I cannot completely release. My father scores 1s in every question above, except one. When it comes to how much this relationship means to me, this relationship gets a 5.

During challenging times in our relationship, I have questioned why we can't get along. I have wondered about his life experiences and what propels him.

In my 20s and 30s, I stayed away from him. Now in my 40s, I selfishly want a relationship with him. I want to know how he is. I want to know where he is, because he is my father. For me, this means he can only have my mobile number. He can't have my address. He may not come to my home. I have established clear boundaries for a relationship in which I feel safe and that allows me to get what I want without sacrificing my wellbeing. If Michael had not agreed to these terms, I was prepared to walk away from this relationship.

* * *

Our relationships should be relatively easy and bring lots of joy more often than not. Yes, things happen, but getting through them doesn't have to feel difficult and lonely. Create relationships that make you feel supported and understood.

As for those relationships that are not good for you but you're not prepared to give up, create boundaries that help you build trust so you can establish connection while feeling protected and safe.

Calm the CHAOS ~ Health and Wellness

The second Element of Living with Purpose is Health and Wellness. This element is about having good mental and physical health and enough energy to get things done daily. Here, you will define what health and wellness mean to you. You will decide how to make your health and wellness what you want it to be, how to create time to do the things that will empower you to achieve and maintain your health and wellness, and how to take care of your internal and your external environments by nourishing yourself when you need nourishment.

According to the American Psychological Association's 2010 Stress in America Study, only 40% of Americans say their health is good. And, while 54% agree that physical activity is critical, only 27% are satisfied with their level of exercise.

We don't move enough, and without realizing it, we make the work harder than it needs to be. When you drink water, eat regularly, and create healthy boundaries, you can engage in life at a new level of excitement, enthusiasm, and appreciation.

Health and wellness are not about looking good. They are about being physically and mentally well. Wellness starts from the inside and works its way out. Being strong mentally and physically is fundamental to fueling your body, mind, and soul for creating total wellbeing.

Like everything else I've shared, this is about *feeling* good. You can't create wellbeing if you don't feel well. Plain and simple. Trying to do so by sheer willpower creates dis-ease in our lives.

You must make decisions that support what you truly desire, and this includes what you eat, what you do, and what you think. Making poor decisions by eating foods that make us tired and feel unwell prevents us from doing the things we need to do to achieve what we want to achieve. When we make good decisions by consuming what fuels our bodies, our moods improve.

If you indulge daily and make poor decisions repeatedly, your body becomes your enemy instead of your ally. This is not to say you cannot enjoy weekend food fests. Just make it a treat, and pair it with proper rest and exercise.

Each day, we make dozens of seemingly small but significant decisions. Long term, the accumulation of these small decisions dictates our chances of acquiring diabetes, heart disease, and cancer.

A 2015 study called "Health, United States," published by the U.S. Department of Health and Human Services, revealed that 48.7% of the population is on regular medication for high blood pressure, migraines, pain, and the like that could be healed with a few lifestyle changes. The side effects of many of these medications take their toll on your health and wellness.

Worse, according to the Surveillance Epidemiology and End Results (SEER) program at the National Cancer Institute (NCI), cancer will affect 1 in 2 men and 1 in 3 women in the United States, and the number of new cases of cancer is set to nearly double by the year 2050.

Worse yet, the CDC.gov – Heart Disease Facts American Heart Association – 2015 Heart Disease and Stroke Update, shows that, since 1984, more women than men have died each year from heart disease.

I don't know about you, but I've already been part of a statistic I don't like, so I'm doing my best to get on the right side of those numbers.

I believe I would not have gotten so sick if I had been mentally and physically well. I experienced illness to the degree I did because I was depleted. I lost my dreams and vision, and I disconnected from everything that created meaning in my life.

When I got sick, I had no fight left. All my power was drained from my body. I had been making mistakes, crying in bathroom stalls, and trying to cover all of it up. I was so ashamed. I didn't know what was happening to me.

I know my story isn't unique. I have listened to different versions of this story, all with the same cast of culprits, for the last five years. When we don't feel good, we don't share and don't talk about it with those closest to us. We don't reach out to those who love us most, and that is a problem. We need to see each other within the courage of our vulnerability. We must share our shame and stop hiding it in the darkness, where its power grows and affects other parts of our lives and bodies.

The point of life is to enjoy living it. If we are in pain, stressed out, and completely fatigued, we must do things differently to create a life worth living.

As we learn how to do better, we must commit to doing better by releasing what we did before knowing what we know now. What happened before doesn't matter. What matters is when you know better, you do better.

When we have a clear understanding of how we want to feel, making healthy decisions about our health and wellness is guaranteed to be so much easier. However, there are certain behaviors that help you achieve total health and wellness.

A Gentle Approach

For decades, I intensely disliked exercise. I tried everything imaginable to get over my hatred. I reframed my thoughts about exercise. I focused on the benefits of looking good and whatever else the "experts" told me to do. But. It. All. Failed. Brilliantly.

It is critical to create health and wellness solutions that you can live with and that fit into the lifestyle you desire.

Moving Forward – Carolina

Carolina is homemaker. Although she takes great pride in the care of her children and husband, she wants to be more than a mother and wife, and she says this longing has made her feel horrible. She reached out to me for help with her weight. Most of her life, she was at a healthy weight, but after having children, she hadn't managed to get fit again. She had the last of their three children five years ago. She was embarrassed to take photos and felt her family was ashamed of her.

Carolina admitted to being an emotional binge eater. She was 50 pounds overweight and felt terrible. She had no drive or energy. It didn't take long to realize that Carolina's self-worth and weight were not separate issues.

While creating her Flight Plan, Carolina discovered that her belief about what it takes to be the perfect mom and wife never allowed her to complain or take time for herself. Even when things were not good, she slapped on a smile and never shared her emotions. Through Carolina's work to create her Flight Plan, she realized the person she has felt most unappreciated and unsupported by is herself.

Nine months after reframing her limiting beliefs, along with installing some new habits and getting rid of others, the excess 50 pounds had come off and, a year later, it has not returned. Her husband tells her he's happy the "old Carolina" is back. Today, Carolina gives herself permission to focus on herself without guilt. She has even started a baby accessory business that she has been dreaming about for years, and she knows she is worth all the health and success she wants in her life.

Workout

Yes, wellbeing includes wellness, and you can't have one without the other. Go for a walk or a run; do yoga, Pilates, or tai chi; swim or dance. What you do doesn't really matter as long as you are moving and enjoying it. For health, make it fun, and do it for at least thirty minutes five times per week and for an hour and a half one day per week.

Eat and Drink Good Stuff

Eating and drinking good stuff at regular intervals during your waking hours will keep you feeling energized and balanced. Do your research, try different meal plans, and select one that supports you and how you want to live.

Drink at least ten glasses of water. Yes, I am very much aware of the recommended eight glasses per day, but I've learned that's not enough. Headaches, bad moods, and reactiveness are all triggered by dehydration, so if you experience any of these, drink up often.

Look Good

Do what it takes to reveal the best version of yourself. Clean up. Put on a nice outfit that makes you feel amazing. Do whatever helps you feel and look your best according to your terms.

For me, this includes waxing where appropriate, dying my grays, putting on a fun, casual, well-fitting outfit, a pair of high-heeled shoes, and handbag to match. It also includes earrings, a necklace, and bracelet. But that's me.

What do you do and wear to look and be your best?

This isn't about being the most gorgeous person in the room; it's about feeling phenomenal when you walk in. It may take a little extra effort, but it's well worth it, especially when you show up with more confidence because you feel good about the way you look.

Sleep

The average person needs between seven-and-a-half and eight-and-a-half hours of sleep, depending on their lifestyle demands. Most of us get by on fewer than six hours per night. We are exhausted and running on fumes. During the time you rest, your body heals and rejuvenates from the wear and tear of living in the Material World.

Be the Priority

I have a gentle approach to health and wellbeing that I'd like to share with you.

For me, health and wellness are about feeling well internally, mentally, and physically. Doctors have told me my healthy weight range is 127 to 154 pounds. My body feels best at 145 pounds.

I feel my current health and wellness are good, and my blood work is phenomenal. My days are full. Because I have lingering issues from The Illness, I am adamant about my morning routine. It fuels me and keeps me focused on what matters each day. I am protective of my time and energy because I don't have the stamina to do everything I want to do and what everyone else wants me to do as well.

Having said that, there are still a few things I can do to achieve the next level of health and wellness for myself, and I want to get better about doing these.

Sometimes I get so wrapped up in my work that, before I know it, it's almost dinner time, and I haven't stopped for a break. Hungry and impatient, I get frazzled easily. Hunger diminishes my self-restraint, so I often snack from the refrigerator while I cook.

Ever been there?

One commitment most of us have trouble making is the commitment to make our health and wellness a priority in our lives.

For many of us, this commitment is as simple as letting go—letting go of things that don't make us feel good.

This isn't just about what you eat. It's also about how you sleep, how you handle your stress, and if you choose to be happy more often than not. It's about loving how you spend your day, so work feels like play. These are not separate things. Together, they make up your health and wellness, and without them, you will never calm the chaos.

If you're lucky, you experience bliss from time to time in your life already, perhaps when you are doing something fun with your family or enjoying big belly laughs with friends or when you're singing your favorite song on the drive home.

Most, however, are not this lucky.

**Seventy-six percent (76%) of women are stressed out;
Sixty-three percent (63%) are exhausted; and
Fifty-four percent (54%) feel guilty. . .**

. . . according to "The Paradox of Declining Female Happiness," a whitepaper published in the American Economic Journal by Betsey Stevenson and Justin Wolfers of the Business and Public Policy Department, The Wharton School at the University of Pennsylvania.

It is now, as you make a commitment to your health and wellness and create a life worth living with passion, purpose, and play, that you must remind yourself what you are doing here, reading this book.

**What does being healthy and well mean to your daily life?
What impact will your new behaviors have on your success?
What talents can you embrace and use to
make this journey more effortless?
What new skills can you acquire to make
this journey more effortless?
Who can you reach out to for support?**

I've been baring my soul to you throughout this book, but this is hard for me to share with you: My entire life, I wanted to be a very slim, 5-foot-7-inch, 24-hour working woman.

But I am not built that way. I am 5 feet 5 inches. I have a broad build and hips that won't quit. Since I'm not growing anymore, I wear three-inch heels every day. I'm not a size 0; I'm a size 10.

I've tried being a vegan and a vegetarian. I've tried liquid and powder diets, with pills and without. I have tried food combining and deprivation. I've even experimented with bulimia to achieve the state of health and wellness others told me I should have.

Thank goodness, I stopped following what people told me to do and started doing the things that felt right for me. By experimenting, I learned that means:

I fall asleep naturally and don't wake up with an alarm.
I give my digestive system a twelve hour rest each day.
I eat meat three times per week.
I drink ginger lemon tea and smoothies most mornings.
I eat two meals per day.
I don't add sugar or salt to my food.
I bust a sweat six times a week for at least thirty minutes.
I limit consumption of bread, sweets, and dairy, including cheese.
I eat what I crave in reasonable amounts. Yes, even the stuff we all agree is not good for us.
I do a coffee enema each week to detoxify my body.

Clearly, I give myself permission to do some of the things that top experts tell us not to do. Some may say I don't have excellent health and wellness. However, I can tell you I have never felt better in my life, health wise.

* * *

My message is this: To acquire the health and wellness you desire, stop listening to what people tell you and find what feels good. Then, do it. Commit to doing what it takes—even the things you don't like—to achieve health and wellness.

SPIRITUAL PRESCRIPTION FOR HEALTH AND WELLNESS

Antidote for not having enough energy to do the things you want to do in a day and for times you feel run down and disengaged from your life.

I fully love and accept myself.
Are you propelled from your bed each morning,
ready, willing, and able to enjoy the day? Or do
you wish you could hide under the covers?

I'm going to ask you to dig deep and face the reality of where your health and wellness are today. Be honest about what you need to do to feel well.

Daily headaches and pain are not normal. Our bodies should not feel as if they are barely getting through the day. Look at your desired lifestyle, and based on what you want to create, be committed to making it your reality.

What do health and wellness mean for you?

We are not all the same when it comes to the demands we make on our bodies.

Do you want to run marathons?
Do you want to climb up the stairs without running out of breath?
Do you want to do a One-Handed Tree Pose at yoga?
Do you want to walk 3 miles in 30 minutes?
Do you want to be able to do things with grace and vibrancy?

What you want to do with your body tells you how you need to take care of it so it will perform as you demand.

What demands do you put on your body?
Is it running around, working, commuting, and taking
care of your obligations and responsibilities?
Is it managing your household and caring for your family's needs
after working a ten-hour day and making a two-hour commute?
Is it focusing on paying your bills and keeping your life
together with the few moments you have left each day?
Or is it all the above?

Where you are now tells you how much work you have to do to
achieve and maintain your health and wellness.

Reflection | How Are You Feeling

Grab your journal and find a quiet place to sit undisturbed for about
40 minutes. Set the mood, so you feel relaxed.

I love to cuddle up with a soft blanket and fluffy pillow, a cup of
tea, and soft music.
It helps me embrace the quiet and release the chaos.

Take a few relaxing deep breaths to center yourself and Tune In.
Once you feel calm, get to work.

While answering the following questions, be honest about where
your health and wellness are today and how supportive your habits
are for the lifestyle you desire. As you do this work, your vision will
become clearer and therefore easier to make your reality.

Let your responses to the following questions and prompts be your
own. Tap into your intuition to lead you to your truth.

What do you want to do each day?
What are your physical goals?
I weigh...

My healthy weight is…
I feel my health and wellness are…
I am great at.…
To achieve the next level of health and
wellness for myself, I want to…

Your answers to these questions tell you where you are now.

When you are done writing, read your responses.

As you close this exercise, reflect on how you feel about what you wrote. Let any emotion or feeling move through you. Don't hold on to judgment or shame. Understand where you are so you can make the transformations that feel good and give you the fuel to take your life to the next level.

Achieve Health and Wellness

Decide what you need to do to feel good and take your health and wellness to the next level. To do that, I want you to stop doing things you don't enjoy, as far as your health and wellness are concerned, and start doing more of the things you do enjoy.

What are you going to do to take your
health and wellness to the next level?
Are you going to drink more water?
Are you going to change the way you eat?
Are you going to do something better than you have been?
What will you do to achieve the health
and wellness you desire?

Be specific about what you will do. This will help you be more mindful of your default habits that do not serve you so you can design habits that do.

Calm the CHAOS ~ Achievement

The third element to Living with Purpose is Achievement. Cultivating the desire to achieve something "more" is a natural feeling most of us have. One of my favorite mentors, Brendon Burchard, speaks about the desire to achieve "more" in two of his books, *The Charge* and *Motivation Manifesto*.

When it comes to achieving our potential, there are a few issues:

We let our beliefs keep us from doing what we want to do.
We let our circumstances prevent us from doing
what we need to do to achieve more.
We let the people in our lives keep us from doing it all.

When I say, "Do the things we want to do," I hope you are putting all your thoughts and energy into creating something truly magnificent and loving. What that means is up to you. I cannot tell you what a magnificent, loving life looks like for you. I can only speak for myself.

For me, a magnificent life means being healthy, wealthy, and happy.

Healthy | I can move and think clearly and do the things I want to do.

Wealthy | I have all of my needs met. I am free.

Happy | I am in a state of joy more often than not.

Our Basic Needs

We all have basic needs. Consciously and subconsciously, we seek to fulfill these needs. According to Human Needs Psychology as taught by Tony Robbins, the six basic needs are universal, and we all try to fill them in varying degrees in our lives.

Certainty | The need for security, stability, and reliability.

Variety | The necessity of change, uncertainty, stimulation, and challenge.

Significance | The need to feel acknowledged, recognized, and valued.

Love and Connection | The need to love and feel loved and to feel connected to others.

Growth | The need to grow, improve, and develop, both in character and in spirit.

Contribution | The need to give, to help others, and to make a difference.

Our quality of life is affected by how we choose to meet these basic needs. We can opt to fulfill our needs in ways that feel good or ways that don't feel good. If the ways we address these needs are not in alignment with our beliefs and values, then we will experience feelings of conflict and discontent. When we align our needs with our highest beliefs and values, not only does life flow with more ease, but we also feel more complete and fulfilled.

Our needs are the drivers of our achievements. If we did not want these things, we would be satisfied with doing nothing and living each day as we did the day before. But the reality is that we are not satisfied. As we move forward in life, we crave achievements big and small, and if we do not honor those feelings, we feel stuck, stagnant, or worse.

There is one thing you can do to define your path for an engaged life that awakens the potential within you: believe you can achieve.

Everything you have experienced until now is the result of real achievements. At some point in your life, you stretched yourself, your skills, your beliefs, and your mental and physical capacities. This stretching brought on greater demands of yourself and your environment. In those moments of deep concentration, your skills and best efforts were put to the test. Your will, strength, and courage were likely pushed to their limits.

During these moments, when the struggle was real and meant something to you, your ability to focus melted away your concerns of time and self-consciousness. As a result, you created and achieved something far greater than you could have conceived, rising above your own limitations, surprising even yourself. This was when real achievement and growth happened. And when it did, I bet you felt more alive and engaged than ever before.

Goals

We all have plenty of things to do in our daily calendars and are busy multitasking, trying to please our bosses, partners, and families, everyone but ourselves. But there's a ginormous difference between achieving and just checking off the boxes on your daily to-do list. This difference is the distinction between surviving and thriving.

Differentiating between your goals and your achievements is important. Your goals are simply things on your to-do list. Nothing in setting a goal demands you show up as your best and highest self. However, challenging yourself to achieve something greater stretches your efforts and abilities.

Busyness is not the same as achievement, just as change is not the same as progress.

We spend the bulk of our lives in a state of busyness, completing those mundane activities that help us maintain where we are: waking up, eating, working, commuting, cleaning, shopping, paying the bills, and taking care of others. Yes, we have to-do lists and checklists aplenty, and we have to manage them all and still remember to do the small things that don't make the lists. If we are honest, really honest, none of these things challenge or push us to achieve anything greater than what we conceived for ourselves ten years ago.

Unfortunately, the chaos, noise, and stress we feel in our Material World are not related to achieving real growth or transformation. Our stress comes from distraction and procrastination. We get too much information, and too many of us spend too much time on unimportant activities and end up in time famines.

Of course, there are plenty of other stressors, and because of them, we feel we cannot take on anymore. Taking care of ourselves or seeking growth seems a luxury saved only for those who "have" time.

You can rise above the mundane murmur of the chaos to achieve more in your life. You can feel more enthusiasm for life, and the way to do it is to conceive a bigger dream for yourself. Achievement is created by choosing fulfilling challenges that bring full engagement and fulfillment in your life with the singularity of focus.

Responsibility

A Spiritual Girl understands that she is in control of her time, her environment, and her destiny. When things happen in her life, she doesn't ask, "Why me?" She asks, "What's next?" She focuses on solutions not problems. She acts and moves forward. She doesn't get stuck in the details of life.

You have a choice to deal with things as you've always dealt with them or to deal with them in a way that serves and honors you and how you want to feel about life.

Every time you decide to let something rock you to your core, you give away your personal power. And when you give away your personal power, you get sick. You don't feel well. Your body tells you, but do you listen? Everything that exists has its shadow and its light. You choose which you will experience and bring into your reality.

Accept responsibility for bringing joy into the world. Accept responsibility for creating your happiness. Accept responsibility for generating love and engagement with others. Accept responsibility for creating a life worth living.

If you have a strong desire to achieve big things for yourself, let nothing deter you from going for it. You alone have the power and responsibility to generate the health, wealth, and happiness you desire in your life. Take it on. Your soul will thank you for it, especially when the going gets tough.

Some people won't feel a strong desire to achieve today, and perhaps never will. If that's you, I just want to ask you to check in and ask yourself why.

If you are in a blissful state and feel no strong urges to do anything more than what you are doing now, embrace that. Your awakening and call to do more will come when you are ready.

If life is chaotic and you don't want to take on anything else, I implore you to calm the chaos and take a more active role in your health, wealth, and happiness. They are yours to be had. Life gets tough and sometimes we can't see past it to the good times that are available for us. But have faith. There is more, lots more, for you to experience. You only have to create it. You have everything you need here to do that. Just take it on, one step at a time.

Dream Bigger

There was a time in my life when I didn't think big. I was happy to survive from one day to the next. I had no time, no money, and no energy. Finally, that day came, the day when I asked myself, "Why don't I think bigger? Why don't I want to be an attorney with my last name on the firm walls? Why don't I want to be Madonna dancing in the limelight? Why don't I want to be Judy Bloom authoring inspirational books?"

I figured it out! I wasn't dreaming big enough. My dreams were limited by my experiences, and all I wanted was to be the twenty-four-hour woman. Without thinking, I had limited my potential. I never dreamed bigger.

Since The Illness, I've learned to step out and dream a bigger dream. Today, my dreams are gigantic and scary, and because of them, life is exhilarating and full.

There are six steps to thinking bigger . . . WAY BIGGER.

How to Think Way Bigger

Step 1 | Run away with your dreams.

It's your turn to dream. Start by finding a tranquil place where you can sit quietly with a few sheets of paper.

Then Tune In, like I described in Chapter 4, and ask yourself:

What would I do to feel fulfilled if there were no barriers in my life?

Next, open yourself up, for 10 minutes, to wondering about what could be possible if you could do anything that you imagine. We often stop ourselves from thinking big because we immediately think, "Who do I think I am?" Or "I'm too old." Or "I'm not enough." It's always something. This is the time to let go of that.

Step 2 | Write down your dreams.

Studies show that when you write out your dreams, you are more likely to make them a reality.

I know this has been the secret of my success—repeatedly. Since I was sixteen, I've written down all my dreams. When I stopped dreaming, my life became stagnant.

Step 3 | Focus on how you want to "feel" when you get to where you want to go.

Unfortunately, this is something most people forget about, and it is one of the most important steps. Focus on the feeling you want, not the photo of what you imagine it will "look" like.

If your dream doesn't make you leap with joy or fill your heart with happiness and your stomach with butterflies, then you know you must find another, bigger dream.

Step 4 | Know what it›s going to take.

For each dream or goal that you have, write out everything it would take to make it happen. This step is about getting clear about what it's going to take to make your dreams your reality.

If it includes learning something new, that's okay. Learn it.

If it includes meeting someone, that's okay. Meet them.

If it includes buying something, that's okay. Buy it.

Write it all out.

There are no limitations to what your action steps may include to successfully achieve what you desire.

Step 5 | Get busy.

Take inspired action, and remember this is not a sprint; it's a marathon. Give yourself time and be patient. Just take one step at a time, knowing you are another step closer to making it happen with each movement forward.

Step 6 | Do it again and again.

Read your goals every day. Hang your list where you can see it. Put your goals on your devices so you can read them anytime. Do so knowing, with each step you take, you are creating the life you've always craved and wholeheartedly deserve. Then, every three to six months, start again by reevaluating your dreams. Make sure you don't end up getting everything you want with nothing you need. Let the things you have lost passion for leave and be open to new inspiration.

That's how I made things in my life happen. As you can see, achieving my goals was never my problem. Committing to my personal dreams and taking care of myself were.

Look at your dreams. It's time to play a bigger game, to dream a bigger dream.

SPIRITUAL PRESCRIPTION TO MAKE YOUR DREAMS YOUR REALITY

Antidote for lack of enthusiasm and dragging yourself out of bed each day because you have nothing to look forward to.

I focus only on my next step and trust that I am being led toward achieving my goals.

Are you doing what's important to you?

You know, those things that make you feel good and really help you live in a way that's rewarding and fulfilling?

If not, it's time to look at what you want so you can put those things on your to-do list. Fill your time with the things that will get you closer to where you want to be.

If you're thinking, "I'm fine, and I'm where I want to be. I'm surviving day to day, doing my work and what I must do. I don't need to do anything else," then I really want you to check in here. Feeling fine or okay about life is the death of living a life of quality and joy.

There is so much more for you to experience than "fine." You are not here to just SURVIVE. You are here to THRIVE.

It's easy to get caught up in everyone else's agenda. The family needs this and that. Someone needs a ride from here to there. But that doesn't mean you can't invest time to take care of your needs.

Let's face it, if you don't take care of yourself and feel delighted and overjoyed with most days of your life, how are you showing up for your family, friends, or the Material World? Consider this to discover those things that will take you from surviving to thriving.

Reflection | Priorities, Priorities

When you have clarity on what matters most, you do more of what you want and less of what you don't. The following process will help you get clear about what matters most so you can focus your time and energy.

11 Steps to Create Priorities that Matter | This process is about *creating* your priorities. Just like clarity, happiness, and energy, you don't find priorities; you create them.

Step 1 | Find a quiet place where you can sit for about ninety minutes. Get eight sheets of paper and title the top of each page:

Business/Career Goals
Financial Goals
Health and Wellness Goals
Spiritual Goals
Family and Friend Goals
Hobbies and Lifestyle Goals
Educational Goals
My Thriving Goals

Step 2 | Before you start to write, take a few, deep breaths and ask yourself, "What do I want to experience now?" Once you feel calm and centered, move on to Step 3.

Step 3 | Write freehand for at least an hour. Write about what you want to achieve from where you are today for the first seven topics above; these are your Topic Lists. Write your hopes and your dreams. Write the things you don't tell anyone else. This is just for you.

Step 4 | When time is up, and only when the time is up, congratulate yourself and look at your Topic Lists. Did you write anything that surprised you? Did you write anything that you have been scared to admit you wanted for yourself? I hope you answered yes. If not, go back and dig deeper.

Step 5 | From each Topic List, select the top 10 things you'd like to achieve. These are your goals for each topic.

Step 6 | Narrow your top 10 goals from each Topic List to three that you want to achieve in the next year to 18 months. We are focusing your field of vision and increasing the likelihood of actually realizing your goals.

Step 7 | Write your top three goals for the next year from each Topic List on the page titled My Thriving Goals. You should now have 21 goals on your My Thriving Goals page.

Step 8 | Now it's time to make some choices because everything on your My Thriving Goals page cannot be a priority at the same time. This dilutes your efforts and makes you feel as if you're spinning your wheels. From the My Thriving Goals page, select the top three goals you will focus on immediately.

Again, congratulate yourself. You have created your priorities. These are the three things you will dedicate and focus all your energy on accomplishing.

Step 9 | For each of the top three priorities you just selected from the My Thriving Goals page, write five milestones that you will achieve to make your goal a reality. These are your tasks.

Step 10 | Assign a time and date to act on these tasks for your milestones.

Step 11 | When you accomplish the three priorities selected in Step 8, look at your My Thriving Goals page again, and select another three.

This, my friend, is how you live a purpose-driven life.

As you read this, you may be thinking that it's easy to say but not so easy to do; I agree. But you must take action to make yourself a priority in your life. I know you can do this. If you don't, who will?

Calm the CHAOS ~ Organization

The fourth element to Living with Purpose is Organization. This is about effectively managing your life by setting yourself up for success.

> When you walk into your home, do you feel
> warm and fuzzy, or frustrated and stressed?
> Do you walk through your doorway with a long,
> drawn-out huff because of all the "stuff"?

A cluttered space is the last thing you want to walk into after a chaotic day in the Material World. If you have too much stuff, the thought of decluttering can feel overwhelming.

Some people are comfortable with knickknacks and photographs on every tabletop, and that's fine. The clutter we are speaking of here isn't about the stuff; it's the emotional baggage attached to the stuff and unfinished business that's standing in your way of achieving the things you want to achieve. This is the stuff that creates the chaos in your life.

Decluttering helps purge all the stuff that takes up more space than it should in your life.

> When you look at your space, does it look loved?
> Cared for? Safe? Comfortable? Warm?

If not, consider:

> What does your space say about how you feel?
> What does it say about your standards?

I am not talking about keeping up with the Joneses. Seriously, who cares about the Joneses? I am talking about living up to your full potential for greatness.

Your home is your haven. It's your safety and refuge from the chaos and noise in the Material World. Your home reflects your current state of being, but if you want, it can also reflect the state of being you desire. Your home should nourish you, as it calls to you after a chaotic and stress-filled day. But, if you are not careful, it can also sabotage you in sneaky and mean ways.

When your space is unloved, it will drain you of all your energy. It will take hold of your attention in small but significant, subconscious ways, causing you to devote less energy to what you want.

Every time you walk into your space and wince at your laundry piled in the corner, that's environmental sabotage.

Every time you decide not to work on that special creative project because you don't have the space or the tools, that's environmental sabotage.

Every time you keep a neighbor on the porch or don't have friends over because you can't face spending the hours it would take to prepare for guests, that's environmental sabotage.

When your space gets in the way of living the life you dream of, that's environmental sabotage.

Moving Forward – Michelle

Michelle is a mortgage broker. She is married and has two adult children and five grandchildren. She grew up very poor but has done amazingly well for herself. She owns a big beautiful home filled with beautiful things. However, when she came to me, she hated going home because the mess was overwhelming. She didn't have enough time to clean as often as she would like, and stuff was everywhere.

Although Michelle is filled with energy, everything she does takes her forever, and she never has all that she needs to finish what she needs to get done. Her home was covered with half-completed projects, as well as mail and newspapers.

The problem for Michelle was that she wanted to keep what she had but needed a better way to manage it so the mess would stop growing. She didn't know where to start.

Creating a Flight Plan has empowered Michelle to take back control of her environment. By thinking through the things that matter to her most, she has reorganized her living space to comfortably fit all the things she wants and to make it easier for her to get rid of things she no longer needs or wants. Previously, this was difficult for her because she grew up so poor; she felt like she had to hold onto everything, even when it served no purpose in her life.

After six months, the house is completely organized, and the excess is gone. Michelle is more aware of how long things take her, so she creates time to clear the mess before it gets out of control. She has cleaned and organized her office, and she credits a boost in her revenue to the Flight Plan; now that she knows what to do and immediately creates the time to do it, she loses fewer leads and closes more deals.

Your Environment

If disorganization lives in your home right now, and you're not sure how to start, start one room at a time. Begin in the room where you spend the most time, the one that affects you the most. That will probably be your living room or your bedroom. Think about:

> What do you need to do and want to do in that space?
> What else would be nice to have in that space?

Then start with a drawer or a shelf and clear it. Remove everything, wipe it down with the appropriate cleanser, and then start putting things in their place. Put only what belongs in that drawer or on that shelf. Put everything else in a basket or a box until you know where you want to put it or what you want to do with it.

Dedicate the Time

You may be thinking, "How much time do I need to dedicate to this?" It depends on your level of disorganization. It could take a few hours to a few days or weeks. Whatever amount of time it takes you, know it is fine. This is not a race. This is not something you are doing for anyone other than yourself.

Do it in the amount of time that feels good to you. If you want to set aside three hours each Saturday until you get it all done, go for it. If you work better in small chunks and want to get it done a bit faster, set aside an hour each day. Stay focused on how you are going to feel and how easy things are going to be to enjoy while you work when your space is organized and you have what you need where you need it.

What's Behind the Clutter

There is a myriad of reasons we keep stuff around. One day, we may have time to read that big stack of books on our nightstands, so we keep piling them up; we might lose that weight, so we don't donate the clothes we can't wear; we may finish that project we started a year ago, so we don't put it away. The fact is that hanging on to far more things than we need makes us feel guilty about what we haven't done instead of motivating us to do it.

We hold onto things because they give us hope. We hope we will read those books. We hope we will lose that weight. We hope we will finish that project. But alas, when it doesn't happen, we beat ourselves up and feel ashamed.

We hold on to things because we think we may need them one day. It's time to understand why you are holding on to what you're holding on to.

By tossing out the old and unworkable, you make way for the new and suitable. A closet filled with clothes you don't use does not invite new clothes that you do wear. A house overflowing with knickknacks you've collected for use someday leaves no space for the things that may truly enhance your life today.

Organize your space in a way that supports your desires.

SPIRITUAL PRESCRIPTION TO SET YOURSELF UP FOR SUCCESS

Antidote for feeling overwhelmed in your environment and as if you don't have the things you need.

I organize my life and my mind.

Now that you know what's causing the environmental chaos, it's time to organize. Before you start, here are a few rules.

Rules to Organize Your Space

Rule 1 | Keep the things that bring you joy and make you feel happy.

Rule 2 | Keep the things that are meaningful and significant to you.

Rule 3 | Keep the things that have a purpose in your life.

Use caution, because there's no reason to be surrounded by things that don't fulfill your needs and wants. When my clients talk about how chaotic their lives are, we often discuss all the clutter in their homes. This is where we start, at the nest.

Reflection | Set Yourself Up for Success

Are you living in environmental chaos?

Do you enjoy being in your space?
Are your rooms cozy and comfortable?
Can you find things you need and want easily?
What doesn't belong that would make
things feel better if they were gone?

Organize in 3 Steps

Now that you know what is not working to help you achieve the success you desire, it is time to set yourself up for success. Here's how you organize in three steps.

Focus on one room at a time. Taking on your whole home is a big job. As you take on each room, consider how you want it to look and how you will use the space. This will help keep you motivated and inspired to finish the job at hand.

Decide what to donate, what to toss, and what to save. Once you have identified items you are going to donate, have a place to store them and take them away as soon as possible. You don't need to wait until everything is done; this will slow your progress. The same goes for the things you are going to toss. Once you've made up your mind, throw them out promptly. Find a permanent place for the items you want to keep. If they will go in a room that has not been decluttered yet, that's okay. Just position the item in an available space; you'll take care of that room when it's time.

Create a space and place for everything. As you think about how you will use each room you're decluttering, decide what kind of areas you need to operate in your home. It's your space. Claim it! If you require places to meditate, write, and work, create them.

Have patience with this process. Don't rush it. The more thought you put into your space, the better it will feel when you are done.

Calm the CHAOS ~ Spirituality

Here we are on the fifth and final element to Living with Purpose: Spirituality. By spirituality, I mean a sense of connection to something bigger than ourselves that involves a search for meaning in life. Spirituality is the connection that keeps you positively expecting epic experiences for yourself and your life, no matter what you are experiencing now.

There comes a time—mine was when I was thirty-eight and I thought I was dying—when you ask yourself, "Is this all there is?" Spirituality helps us cope this and helps us be happy with the answers to those questions we ask later in life. Remember, those questions I talked about before:

> Did I matter to anyone other than myself?
> Did I love boldly and openly?
> Did I truly live up to my best and highest potential?

Because of what we experience some days, spirituality is hard for most to master and understand. However, if we can't get here, are we creating a life worth living?

To be clear, the spirituality I'm referring to is not about blindly believing in any theories or stories that your personal experience cannot support. It's all about going within by creating a practice of processing your thoughts and allowing your intuition to guide you as you align with your truth. When you do this, the meaning and purpose of your life become apparent.

Spirituality is taking the time to look within with a quiet mind and gentle heart to connect to your higher loving self.

When I started my "Spiritual Journey," I didn't realize what I was doing. I felt raw and vulnerable. After The Illness, I wanted to know why I survived. I needed my suffering to have meaning.

Most people are happy to endure the struggle and move on with their life. But I needed to know why. I needed to know why I made it out of that bed and my friend Jenny did not.

Jenny is one of my soul sisters. We met shortly after I moved to Orlando. She anchored me while my life was chaotic. She'd take me to the beach with the kids to enjoy the day. She'd help me relax in the evening while we chatted about our days. I was a working mom, and she stayed home with her boys.

Just before Christmas 2010, I got a call from Rich, Jenny's husband. He had news that changed our lives. Jenny had a brain tumor. The message in our call was that the doctors were going in, and then we would know more.

So there I was with whatever (we found out it was neurological Lyme disease in 2012) and had no idea what was going on, and there she was, diagnosed, and she knew what was going on. Was The Illness really in my head?

Was Jenny's circumstance my wake-up call to start my healing by digging deeper? I had to know why: why did I have nothing, according to all the doctors, yet I felt as if I was dead? Why was Jenny diagnosed with something horrific yet felt so alive?

Jenny had her operation; it was brain cancer. She lived for almost 30 months after her diagnosis. And, again, I asked why? Why am I alive, and why has she passed on? I have to believe it's because she fulfilled her life's mission, and I have yet to fulfill mine.

This is why I share my message. Because in healing my body, I had moments that felt like I was here to do more. Spirituality pulled me through.

Truth

It may seem to be a radical idea: that all humans, regardless of who we are, where we're from, or what our backgrounds are, "should" be spiritual. But what if I told you that that's not enough? What if I told you we NEED to be more spiritual simply to be happy and psychologically healthy? The idea that human beings need purpose and direction in life is not novel, but so few understand this at a conscious level.

Spirituality is not black and white. There is a large gray area where most people fall. Maybe they believe in God or a higher purpose in a vague sense, or maybe they just think everything happens for a reason, but that's the extent of it. They don't practice any form of spirituality or work on themselves for enlightenment.

Spirituality relates to almost any kind of meaningful activity, personal growth, or joyful experience. Traditionally, spirituality refers to a process of re-formation of the personality, but there is no real definition of spirituality. After World War II, spirituality and religion became disconnected. A new conversation has developed in which mystical and esoteric traditions and Eastern religions are being blended to reach the true self by self-disclosure, free expression, and meditation.

I am a baptized Roman Catholic, but I haven't practiced my religion for twenty years. I do find comfort in the traditions, things like praying the Rosary, Our Father, Hail Mary, and confession. I also meditate, keep blessed crystals in my bra, journal, and honor saints and ascended spirits. I also firmly believe God lives in me and every other human being and is ever-present in everything living. I imagine tethers energetically pulling us toward Him. It's what connects us.

The beauty of spirituality is that once you commit to it, a world of synchronicity and new experiences opens for you. The moment you decide that spirituality is "for you," it's as if the doors of enlightenment swing open and you finally start to see the Material World through eyes of love.

The truth is, all beings are inherently spiritual. Some just don't know it.

The longer you practice spirituality, the more devoted you become. Understand that it is a way of life, not a hobby or passing interest, the more it gives back to you.

Spirituality helps you lean back, chill out, and enjoy the ride of your lifetime.

An issue no one speaks about is that most people don't feel connected to why they exist. They are sleep-walking through their days, hoping that everything works out for them in the long term, accepting what life throws at them without will or intention, letting someone else decide how much health, wealth, and happiness they deserve.

To live spiritually is to live in alignment with your values, beliefs, and loving desires. We are all in this collective experience and responsible for sharing our brilliance for the greater good. Each of us is connected and here to play a critical role in the heath, wealth, and happiness of our Material World. However, the chaos and noise distracts us from the truth by way of alcohol, drugs, overwork, toxic relationships, toxic food, overeating, and many other forms of life's harmful chaos.

We need spirituality.
It connects us to our purpose and gives us direction.

No matter where we fall on the happiness meter, there is always another level of love and engagement of living when we connect to our spirituality. And just when we think it can't get any better, it does.

I shared the story of my friend Jenny with you. She passed away from terminal brain cancer and was an atheist most of her life. She firmly held her belief that our sole purpose is to live and die and that there is nothing before or after. However, from the time she was diagnosed until her passing, Jenny thought a lot about life. We regularly spoke about spirituality.

Jenny passed away when she was forty-three. She lived a lot of life in that short time, including the loss of her son Arick. She struggled with his passing and, at first, saw this tragedy as confirmation of there being nothing more to us than flesh and blood. She suffered tremendous pain until she asked her end-of-life questions. What if she believed in a higher power? What if she believed there was something more to our lives?

She came to me, feeling like a fraud because she now believed in the love and power of spirituality, which she defined as God, all-knowing and all-consuming. Jenny thought the timing of her belief and faith in God was a bit too convenient and called herself a hypocrite. Now that she was going through these trials and tribulations of losing one of her sons and now her life, she wondered why she blamed the lack of God as the reason for her suffering. She never gave God credit when things were going well. I counseled her on the fact that there is no time limit or judgment when it comes to the love of God or source or whatever you want to call your Inner Guidance. It comes when it comes.

I share this with you so you will give yourself permission to explore your spirituality without limitations or judgment. This is your journey. Let nothing keep you from stepping out fully to discover what spirituality means to you.

What is important is that you develop a practice to connect with your inner self, your highest and most loving desires to create a life worth living.

Self-Forgiveness

Lots of things keep us from being who we desire to be and from feeling what we desire. As issues arise, we need to work on them. Many of our internal struggles come from the need to forgive ourselves and fully accept responsibility for where we are now. As you mend your fences and heal old wounds, remember forgiveness.

When we talked about Connection, I shared what forgiveness is and isn't so you can release and heal old wounds that involved others. Sometimes, we forgive those we fault for our wounds, those who abused us in one form or another, those who hurt us intentionally, those who hurt us unintentionally. But when do you forgive yourself for any part you took in the hurt?

I forgive. I completely forgive. I forgive those who have hurt me. I forgive myself for not trusting. I. Forgive. Myself.

I honor you for doing this work. This is the tough work. This is the work that causes true transformations in your character and, hence, transcendence.

Release the Past

Have you ever caused a hurt so deep you still don't forgive yourself for it? Even if it's been years, each time you see the person you hurt, your heart starts beating faster, and your stomach knots up with fear and emotion.

When we hurt the people we love, hopefully, we find a way to apologize and make things right with them. However, we don't go through the same process with ourselves. If the pain you caused is almost unbearable, and each time you see the person—even if they forgave you—you still feel shame and hurt, it's time to go inward to forgive yourself.

I beat myself up for having a baby when I was sixteen. This hurt my mother and my family. Over time, they forgave me, but it would take decades for me to realize how angry I was at myself. My anger and resentment kept me from experiencing all the wonderful things that were happening in my life. Nothing I did was ever right or perfect enough. I punished myself continuously because of it.

Remember Denise from *Moving Forward*, who at sixteen gave her daughter up for adoption? She went through the same type of torment, until she forgave herself.

We are all worthy and deserving of forgiveness. Forgiveness is a process that involves transforming an emotion and feeling about the person who does the wrong—in this case, ourselves. Realize there is no way to maintain a healthy relationship, especially with yourself, without forgiveness.

5 Steps to Self-Forgiveness

Here is a process I developed for self-forgiveness. I hope it inspires you to explore forgiveness for yourself so you can fully heal and release hurt and resentment.

Step 1 | Dig deep. Look inward to reflect on what you are feeling about the hurt you committed. Ask yourself, "Was the hurt accidental or intentional?"

Step 2 | Let yourself off the hook. Consider what forgiveness is and isn't. Then make a conscious decision to forgive yourself. Ask yourself, "Can I forgive myself for my part?"

Step 3 | Understand "why." Reflect on the situation to take responsibility for your actions, and your actions alone. Realize you do not have control of other people. Ask yourself, "What could I have done differently?"

Step 4 | Find the lesson. Learn from your experience so the next time you encounter a similar situation, you respond from a place of love and don't react in fear. Ask yourself, "What did I learn, and what wisdom can I gain from this experience?"

Step 5 | Let it go. Let go of the pain and stop wishing things could have happened differently. The whole purpose of living is to grow, so do that. Be open to the lessons and carry your wisdom as your badge of honor.

If you have a past hurt or wrong that you were forgiven for, yet you still experience shame or guilt, grab a journal or a few sheets of paper and write about it as you go through the process to self-Forgiveness, and forgive yourself.

Meditation

Let's talk about meditation for a stronger connection to our Inner Guide. In Chapter 4, where I shared the Peace Practice, I talked about the benefits of mediation. It's worth mentioning again how beneficial mediation is to quality living and connecting to your Inner Guide.

You don't learn from your experiences.
You learn by reflecting on your experiences.

Here's a simple meditation you can do anywhere, anytime.

Get comfortable. Rest your hands on your lap. If you can, play soft music or listen with headphones to soothing sounds like running water. Consider keeping a notebook or journal and pen at hand for any notes or inspired ideas that come during your meditation.

Breathe in and out as you feel comfortable.

Let your thoughts drift in and out. Don't hold on to them. Let them come and go. If something comes up that you don't want to forget, write it in your journal. Many people believe the ideas and thoughts that come through meditation are divinely guided and inspired.

Continue this cycle of breath until your mind feels clear and uncluttered.

After clearing your mind, free-think, or if you have a topic in mind, focus on that but avoid dead end, angering, and solution-less subjects. Focus on issues for which you are confident you can find new ground and progress. Another option is to look into your life or your inner self and think about what's going on right now—anything that will help you focus and see helpful pictures or thoughts.

When you are done with your meditation, journal or draw, if you feel inspired.

Gratitude

Gratitude is a special tool we can use every day, especially in turbulent or emotional times. When life is in chaos, we must still show up with grace, faith, and gratitude. Practicing your Spirituality will help keep you in a place where you can look at the Material World through eyes of love.

You cannot be of service when you feel as low as the person you want to help. You want to be of service by offering a hand out of honor, not pity. By connecting to your Inner Spirit, you connect to your courage to serve from a place of strength.

The best time to give gratitude for what's around you is when you're stuck on what's going on and not working for you. Focus on what you want to feel and think about what will get you closer to that goal. Don't try to find the good in what has you stuck, find the good in what is working for you. True gratitude helps us see our situation through a different lens, in a settled, more rational way that spurs our creativity to find a solution.

We are hardwired to be grateful; however, we lose touch with that part of our lives. In fact, I was taught that expressing gratitude and happiness may actually "jinx" us and can change any good fortune to bad.

Dr. Robert Emmons, author of ***Thanks! How Practicing Gratitude Can Make You Happier***, says there are three stages to giving gratitude.

Three Stages to Giving Gratitude

Stage 1 | Recognizing what we're grateful for.

Stage 2 | Acknowledging it.

Stage 3 | Appreciating it.

Sounds simple, right? But like many other things, it isn't easy for everyone. Like any skill you want to master, gratitude takes practice.

Deepen Your Spirituality

There are many ways to deepen your connection to your Inner Spirit. I suggest you do research or seek out a spiritual group.

Do research. Research the native religions/spiritual beliefs of the people who lived in your country in the past. Check the internet and the library for more information on such old religions for an alternative spiritual view. The spiritual beliefs of your ancestral roots may speak to you about your family history.

Seek out a spiritual group. Go with a friend. This can be any size group. Have some questions in mind beforehand, and ask them at an appropriate time.

* * *

Spirituality is a personal and sacred practice. Explore your Spirituality in a way that honors how you want to feel about your days and life.

SPIRITUAL PRESCRIPTION FOR SPIRITUALITY

Antidote for feeling unfulfilled and unhappy, when you don't find the joy in your work, and family feels more like a burden than a blessing.

I am grateful for all that I have and all that I will receive.

In our day-to-day lives, with all the noise and chaos of the Material World, it's easy to lose connection to how amazing life is.

There are so many reasons we lose connection:

> Life blends in and out of exhausting, stressed-out days.

> An extraordinary event happens, and you deal with it by checking out.

> Our bodies break down and remind us of our humanity.

But that doesn't mean you cannot connect to your Inner Guidance.

Know there is no life circumstance too small to shift your world from high to low or low to high. It's all about how you respond and how you allow it to affect you.

5 Ways to Let Gratitude Take the Lead

Letting gratitude take the lead every day is a simple way to keep from disconnecting; it opens you to your Inner Guide so you remember to honor your health, wealth, and happiness.

Be mindful. As I have discussed, mindfulness is being aware of why you feel the way you feel. Mindfulness is so important that I speak about it in most of my talks. If you need a refresher, I led with it in the section titled "Where Do You Want To Go," where I shared the 3 Principles of a Thriving Mindset.

Find one thing to be grateful for. You can make this as simple as you like. What's important is that you create a process that feels good. When I started my Gratitude Practice, I kept a Gratitude Journal. However, since 2014, I've created Gratitude Pages. At the beginning of each year, I simply grab a legal-size sheet of paper from my printer and write: "(YEAR) I am grateful for . . . " and pin it to my bulletin board. Each day, I find one thing to be grateful for and write it on my Gratitude Page. After just a few weeks, so many things are listed that just looking at it gives me a mental boost. My Gratitude Page gives me a sense of pride and meaning that swells within me every time I see it.

Switch your thoughts. If something you are experiencing is affecting you negatively, shift your thoughts and find something that makes you feel more grateful. It can be anything from your circumstances to the weather. Using the weather, here's an example of how I do this.

I don't enjoy cold weather, and saying, "don't enjoy" is an understatement. I live in Florida where cold should not be an issue; however, I have discovered the hotter it gets outside, the more arctic stores and restaurants keep their inside temperatures. Therefore, I am always freezing, exactly the opposite of why I came to Florida. I used to complain about it. Now, I always carry a sweater or a wrap and focus on the comfort I feel when I wrap myself up. The temperature no longer infects my thoughts or my mood with things that feel bad.

Stop complaining. Complaining serves no purpose and makes you feel worse than you should. Talking about what is going on in a way that focuses on finding answers and solutions serves to help you feel better. When we complain, we fuel our negative emotions and improve nothing. Focus on the solution, not the problem.

Learn from your challenges. We are growth-seeking beings and are here to experience everything life has to offer. Our challenges teach. When you're going through a rough time, ask yourself, "What am I learning? What will I be grateful for when this is done?"

Reflection | Give Gratitude

There's a reason why so many people talk about gratitude to feel good. It works. There was a time when giving gratitude was hard for me. I must have said I am thankful for air every day for a month before I thought to be grateful for my family. I just couldn't get there.

Give gratitude daily for what you appreciate. Lots of people say it should be three things a day, but I want you to do what feels good. You can also do a rampage of appreciation each day where you say all the things you appreciate in that moment about a particular person, thing, or situation.

Again, feel your way through to what feels good for you, but do this. It helps you stay tuned into the joy in your life.

Chapter 6

Live with Play

"Success is never an accident. It is always the result of a commitment to be your best, deliberate planning, and focused effort." ~Carmen M. Perez

It's finally time to pull everything together to create a Flight Plan that will empower you to soar to new heights.

I know we took the long way to get here, but I don't believe you should run your days with what others tell you is right for you. You can only get so far when you don't do what feels good and right to you. I have given you the guidelines and, hopefully, you have done the work to define what is going to take you to that next level of health, wealth, and happiness.

This is how you achieve true success. Success does not come at the cost of huge sacrifice. It comes as an abundance of success in all areas of your life.

At some point, we learned that we are not supposed to enjoy play as adults. Work is serious business, and play is not allowed. As a result, we make ourselves too busy and decide there are more important things to do. As it turns out, few things are more important to your wellbeing than play.

In fact, when we see an adult playing, we often laugh at them, say they're crazy, or judge them and think they need to grow up. We may make fun of them behind their back and, worse, stop taking them seriously.

Being an adult does not mean we cannot play. In fact, it means we can give ourselves permission to play more.

I developed The 7 Keys of Effective Productivity so we can do the things we need to do faster and create each day to feel more like play, and less like work.

Living with Play is my favorite and last critical component of the Flight Plan. To Live with Play, we must reclaim our time and energy by focusing on what empowers us to achieve success in our lives without sacrificing our health, wealth, and happiness.

Once I learned to see the Material World through eyes of love and focus on what matters most by calming the CHAOS, creating a life worth living was easy to embrace. The 7 Keys offer a practical and more conscious way of doing things.

It is time for us to move forward faster while taking life one day at a time. This sounds contradictory, but when we reclaim our time, we can enjoy more of the magic and synchronicity life has to offer. As you invest your time in the Material World, the 7 Keys will guide you so you can effectively and efficiently create a life worth living.

How to Quiet the Noise and Calm the CHAOS

As I shared how to Live with Purpose with connection, health and wellness, achievement, organization, and spirituality, you probably thought, "Okay, great. How do I do that?" I know, with your daily obligations and responsibilities, it may seem like Living with Purpose is a far-off destination. What I am about to share with you will empower you to get closer to that magical destination without all the frustration and overwhelm that is usually involved in creating a life where each day feels more fulfilling and meaningful.

I firmly agree with George Bernard Shaw when he said,

> *"We don't stop playing because we grow old;*
> *we grow old because we stop playing."*

We must stop wasting precious time trying to attain perfection, taking control of everything just because we can, and doing things we really don't want to. We must create time for the things that bring us fulfillment and meaning, and they don't have to be separate from the work we do. Society has told us that play is a luxury we cannot afford.

The further we go in our life journey, the more distracted we get by life and things that don't make us feel good. Life is not something you survive or need to suffer through. You are meant to thrive. Life is amazing, and you are supposed to take in all that life has to offer.

It's time to tear down the walls that you've built being the person you were told to be and create a life you love being the person you know deep down inside you truly are. You don't have to wait for your circumstances to change or to get over something. Start now.

Invest Your Time

The 7 Keys will show you how to do what you need and want to do with more play, bringing more impact to achieving your desires and enthusiasm for everything you do. I write this knowing full well how difficult it is, but it is a must to make the most of your every day. Realize it's a challenge because we have been trained to make a choice between work and play, but it's time to change that.

Play connects you with who you really are and the things you enjoy that fulfill you. Researchers say that the more we absorb ourselves in the joy of what we are doing, the happier we are. In 2015, the Society for Human Resource Management's HR News webpage reported results of "The It Pays to Play Study," commissioned by HR Cloud Software Company. The study revealed that play increases performance and sparks creativity. Play helps us align with our deepest needs and live in the moment. Your ability to enjoy play is directly linked to a positive mood and a happier life because it buffers the effects of stress on your immune system and amplifies your vitality.

Set the intention to bring more play into your day. What's the sense of achieving success if you don't feel successful?

Create More Opportunity

Somewhere along our journey, we took on the belief that we must take life seriously, so we have. But I want you to challenge that belief. Create ways to infuse your day-to-day routine with play, so you don't sacrifice your health, wealth, and happiness while doing the things you need to do and want to do.

There's no reason for you to wait until you finish that big project, make that money, or buy that house to create a life worth living. You owe it to yourself, those around you, and the Material World, to create a life worth living now. Otherwise, what's the point?

Enjoy the process of conquering the struggles by celebrating your successes. They make life all that it is.

Admit it.

When you look back at some of your greatest challenges, do you realize what gifts were left behind?

What did you learn?
Who did you bond with?
How did it change your life?

These are the things we must carry with us. The purpose in our problems is not the pain; it's the preference. Without understanding what we want and don't want, we cannot gain preference or clarity on what we want for ourselves.

Create a daily reminder to yourself to Live with Play. Life isn't all about work and making money, which is why I created the 7 Keys to Effective Productivity, not so you can do more, but so you can play more.

Putting The Keys to work in your life will infuse your days with passion, purpose, and play. Take on your challenges, and everything else you need and want to get through in your life, with clarity and focus, faster and easier.

You don't need to fill every minute of every day with mundane tasks and numbing social schedules.

You don't have to push and forge your way through every day to get what you want.

You don't have to suffer exhaustion, guilt, or stress either.

These are illusions cast upon us by the chaos and noise of the Material World. Now that you know what you need to do to thrive and live with Passion, Purpose, and Play, let me show you how to get it all done.

Bringing It Together

Between what you need to do and what you want to do, you probably feel that you don't have time left for creating deeper and more meaningful connections, for improving your health and wellness, for achieving the things you've been dreaming about, for organizing your life to suit how you want to live, or for bringing more spirituality into your life.

I get it. Trust me, I do. I didn't leave time for these things until I didn't have a choice. But you know now what I didn't know then, and that alone will make it easier for you. When you stray from your chosen path, you will feel it because of your awareness, which will empower you to bring yourself back to your chosen path.

The Keys

The Keys are how you live with Passion, Purpose, and Play. They will help you accomplish all the things you have consciously decided you want and need to do. They will help you achieve true success in life, if your definition of success is achieving your deepest and truest desires without the filters the Material World places on them. Using The Keys is how I wrote this book. With The Keys, I created a well-known and successful tattoo studio, a travel business, and a personal business success mentorship practice.

The Keys empower you to reclaim your time. With them, you can do the things you need and want to do, stay on track so you can do more, and save time while making an impact on your success with the quality of your health, wealth, and happiness.

Let's talk about what's going on now and why only 7% of the population has figured out how to achieve and maintain their wellbeing.

Time Management

We've all heard people say, "I need to learn to manage my time."

Do you think this way too?

If so, I hate to tell you this, but you can't manage time. We all have exactly the same amount of time in the day: 24 hours. No one gets to extend them. No one gets to buy spare minutes. This is one of those non-negotiable situations, yet I hear people say this all the time.

What we can manage is our effectiveness.

For the last five chapters, I've shared what it takes to achieve total wellbeing and enjoy the synchronicity that you create by living in complete alignment. It's a lot, but don't you owe it to yourself to give this life your all? I think you do. By developing supporting behaviors, habits, and systems, you create more ease and flow in your life.

Imagine a world in which everyone lived in alignment with Passion, Purpose, and Play and with optimal health, wealth, and happiness.

Imagine if everyone was driven to live to their best and highest desired potential by integrating their desired levels of connection, health and wellness, achievement, organization, and spirituality.

Wouldn't that be phenomenal?

There would be no anger, guilt, or resentment. Everyone would bring their joy, vigor, and vitality to live the life their soul intended.

Reclaim Your Time

Do you feel you are working as hard and as efficiently as you can?
Are you wondering what to tackle first
because there's too much to do?
When you have a full plate, are you saying
"yes" when you really mean "no"?

You are not alone. The study I shared previously, "The Paradox of Declining Female Happiness," revealed that about 80% of us feels guilty, exhausted, and/or stressed out. The book **Wellbeing: The Five Essential Elements**, written by Tom Rath and Jim Hartner, confirmed what 93% of us feel but don't speak about, which is that there never seems to be enough time to do the things we need to do, let alone the things we want to do.

My whole life, I have understood how to get the work done. It's my brilliance. When it comes to strategizing and execution, I can see right through the disorder that slows our thinking, that keeps us from feeling free, and I can create a plan that gets things done.

I discovered this ability while managing hundreds of real estate closings when I worked as a commercial real estate paralegal. I also used it to help my husband create his tattoo business. I put it to work again when I created sojourns and the sales funnels to sell them out.

Then, I realized the power of this skill as I worked with conscious, service-based businesses and entrepreneurs. Not only can I help them achieve more success by teaching them how to create growth, marketing, and management systems, but I also help them enjoy more of the success they have created through my knowledge of a Thriving Mindset, Calming the CHAOS, and The Keys.

There's nothing I can do to get you out of the work it will take. But having a guide will prevent you from squandering your precious time and will help you stay on the right path to enjoy your journey with more ease.

No more settling.
No more mediocrity.
No more just getting by.

Effective Productivity

Effective productivity is the ability to make a deep impression on what you are creating. What we create is amazing for us and for everyone around us, because, as we create a life worth living, we give others permission to do the same.

The Keys help you take your days from surviving to thriving. I want you to go from, "I'm happy to just get through the day" to "I can't believe I got it all done and I feel great." That's the difference, babe. You want to feel good, don't you? So, let's go for that.

The Keys are how we do it. After the summaries below, we will go through them in detail, one at a time, so you can Live with Play, do more in less time, and do more of what makes you feel good. As you put The Keys to work, you will reclaim your time, calm the chaos, and positively transform the way you experience your world.

Key 1 | Thoughtfulness

Generally, we don't think deliberately about who we want to be, where we want to be, or what we want to do. We live unconsciously, bullied and pushed by the chaos of the Material World. Through the Key of Thoughtfulness, you will no longer live by default, bending and flexing to meet The Others' definition of success and happiness. You will take charge of your thoughts and of how you show up in the Material World.

Thoughtfulness connects you to what you truly want to achieve so you can focus on what will create your life worth living. Only when you know where you are and where you want to go can you move forward with real direction.

Key 2 | Regulate

The second Key, Regulate, is how we keep out what doesn't support us and, instead, let in what will. You will determine, with amazing clarity, what you must do to set yourself up for success. Without clarity, we cannot know what must be true to make our dreams reality.

We don't often make a direct impact on the quality of our lives because we are distracted and haven't found a way to bust through the blocks to achieve the success we desire. This Key will empower you to invest your time doing what matters and creating boundaries that honor your wellbeing.

When you know what's important to you at a deeper level, knowing what to do becomes simpler.

Key 3 | Assign

When you get to the third Key, you will know what you want to do and need to do to achieve success. This Key puts pen to paper, actually creating the schedule that will drive your days and strategizing to live with Passion, Purpose, and Play. Being enlightened about your true desires makes the practical action part of planning your Flight Plan more powerful.

Through this Key, you will set yourself up for success, so you make empowering decisions and do the things that will take you one step closer to where you want to be.

While there is a freedom and lure to flying by the seat of your pants—which I recommend doing from time to time—that is not a way to live a purpose-driven, fulfilled, and meaningful life. By thoughtfully designing a Flight Plan that highlights your brilliance, character, and desire, you can see the practical action steps necessary to bring your deepest desires to life.

Key 4 | Vigilance

Keys 1 through 3 will build your momentum and give you a place to focus your energy. You know what you want, you know what to do, and you know when you are going to do it. Key 4 | Vigilance will keep you moving with inspired action, so you do the things you say you are going to do when it's time to do them.

One of the essentials to getting what you want is taking action when it's time to take action. Creating your Flight Plan is just the first step. The next crucial step is taking focused action when you say you will.

Key 5 | Extract

The power of this Key will help you look at those things keeping you from achieving what you set out to do, so you can clear your path to live to your true desired potential. So much information comes to us on a daily basis that it's dumbfounding. The problem with this is we don't know what to do with it all.

Through processes, strategies, and systems that you will develop through this Key, you will disintegrate the piles, real and virtual, that distract you from doing what you set out to do.

Key 6 | Learn

As you take on the Flight Plan, things will expose themselves that you may not be prepared to deal with. That's okay. Life is about learning, and Key 6 | Learn is about finding ways to take your lifestyle to the next level. You are going to stay fluid and open to new opportunities you've never dreamt, and you will expand your skills.

This is where you take an honest look and seek out information and knowledge that will help you achieve the success you desire. Too often, we allow not "knowing" to get in the way of achieving our deepest desires. Trust that everything is figure-out-able.

Key 7 | Self-Love

Self-love is the most important yet the most neglected part of creating a life worth living. When we don't care for our needs, how can we possibly show up as our highest best self? We end up living in the comfort of running around like chickens trying to tackle our to-dos.

Self-Love gives you an opportunity to relax, rejuvenate, and rejoice. This is the one thing we consider a luxury, but it definitely is not. Key 7 | Self-Love gives you permission to be, to rest, and to celebrate. Through this Key, you will create routines that reward your body, mind, and soul with the adoration, affection, and appreciation they deserve for their faithful service to you.

* * *

The Keys will empower you to live in alignment and keep on your path to creating a life worth living. By using The Keys to guide you through your days, you will execute living with Passion and Purpose in a way that supports how you want to live to achieve success without compromising your health, wealth, and happiness.

Beautiful Soul, you have a lot to look forward to.

Let's take on The Keys, one at a time.

SPIRITUAL PRESCRIPTION FOR LIVING IN ALIGNMENT

Antidote for feeling like you have no control over your happiness or your choice.

I live in alignment with my values, beliefs, and desires.

Do you feel like you are in a constant state of motion but aren't getting anything significant done throughout the day?

Here are The Keys and the questions that will help you stay on your path so busyness no longer rules your life. This is how we use The Keys to think through incidental challenges we experience in life.

Thoughtful
Be thoughtful about what you want and how
you want to show up in the world.
**Is what you want to do getting you
closer to where you want to be?**

Regulate
Know what you want and need to do to get there.
**Is what you want to do in alignment with
what you want for yourself?**

Assign
*Decide when you will do the things that will
impact and support your success.*
Is this worth investing time in?

Vigilance
Do what you say you're going to do when you say you're going to do it.
Do you have the energy to do it?

Extract
Get what you want from the chaos and get rid of everything else.
Will this feel supportive or sabotaging?

Learn
Open your mind to accept new information that
will take you where you want to be.
Is there something to learn from this?

Self-Love
Be your greatest fan and allow yourself to be your greatest priority.
Does what you want to do feel fulfilling?

Ask yourself the questions, be honest with the answers, and live in alignment with what you truly and deeply desire.

Reflection | Go from Surviving to Thriving

Work through The Keys to go from surviving to thriving and relieve that all-too-familiar feeling of being stuck, not knowing where to go or what to do next, when you know something does not feel right but cannot put your finger on it.

Think through the issue you are struggling with so you can be led to your personal, "right" solution. This is not a one-size-fits-all effort. We all want different things at different levels. What abundance means to me may not be what it means for you, and until you uncover your higher desires, nothing will ever feel right or good as you move through your days.

Whether it's considering a new job, getting a divorce, moving from one home or state to another, or going out for drinks after work, go through The Keys sequentially, and you will be led to do what is right for you, without guilt or regret.

While at times you may feel selfish, know you are not. Serving your highest good helps your family, friends, and the Material World. Imagine if we all lived this way. What could be possible for the Material World and how we live in it?

When you feel too busy, ask yourself:

Is your busyness closing the gap between where you are and where you want to be, or is it keeping you from achieving your dreams and getting what you want?

Think through The Keys to start doing the things that make a bigger impact on helping you get what you want and achieve success.

How I Use The Keys to Go from Surviving to Thriving

I thought it would help for you to read how I apply The Keys to my life and the situations that come up. Here's an example.

I am agoraphobic, meaning I have a fear of being in crowds, public, and open spaces. This fear keeps me home, sometimes for weeks at a time. I know this seems strange for someone who is a motivational speaker and travels the world to share her message. I wish I could explain why I have this fear, but I really don't know.

There are times when I am supposed to go out, and I start panicking. Horrible thoughts come to my mind about all the things that could happen as a result of my stepping out of the house. I know this is irrational, and most of the time I am successful at getting myself through this struggle by using The Keys.

This is how I go through the steps when we need groceries for the house.

Thoughtful | Someone needs to go grocery shopping. Do I want to go or shall I send one of the kids? There are always so many people at the store, but I really want to get the things I want from the grocery store myself. When I send other people, I forget to put things on the list and don't get to make the things I want. I want to see what new foods are on the market and what I can experiment with. I should go myself. I want to go. It will be good for me to get air, and I want to be more social, so I will go.

Regulate | What do I need from the grocery store? Let me make a list of everything I want to eat so I can get what I need to make it. I don't want to forget anything or not have enough of something I want.

Assign | When will I go to the store? Is there someone who could go with me? Let me go to the grocery store on Sunday morning. I'll ask Miggie, my daughter, if she can go with me. That will make me feel more secure. If I go early, there won't be too many people there.

Vigilance | Is everything I need where I need it so I can go when it's time? I'll double-check the list I made in my digital grocery application. I'll also put my grocery bags where I won't forget them.

Extract | Is there anything else I need to do Sunday that may keep me from going to the grocery store? I double-check my schedule and prepare my things so I can go without any last-minute effort that could stall me and give me time to rethink leaving.

Learn | Is there anything else I can do simpler or faster to prepare to go to the grocery store so it doesn't take so much mental energy? When I get back from the store and put things away, I think through how I felt and if my adventure was successful. Then I think about anything I could do to make my adventure easier.

Self-Love | What is my reward for going to the grocery store? I have everything I need and was able to get things I didn't put on the list. It felt good going outside, and I could treat myself with a drink from my favorite café.

This may seem trivial, but if you have any fears or situations you face on a regular basis, seeing how I get through mine will hopefully help you use the Steps to Go from Surviving to Thriving to get through yours.

You can use The Keys to Go from Surviving to Thriving to consider moving, taking a new job or promotion, getting a divorce, buying that designer handbag, or going on vacation. Use The Keys for anything and everything you want to thrive through.

Key 1 | Thoughtfulness

This Key requires thoughtfulness about who you are, how you behave, and how you contribute in the Material World.

Not until I took care of my wellbeing did I see what that did for those around me. My family was used to me being a high-strung perfectionist. When I started practicing this Key, they felt more relaxed and able to approach me. They sensed more peace and calm in our home.

At first, this realization shamed me. I even felt guilty. My perfectionism was the way I dealt with the chaos in the Material World. Everything needed to be perfect: perfect clothes to play the part of the twenty-four-hour woman at work, perfect hair to go with the persona I was building, perfectly kept home and matching family to go with the identity I was working so hard to achieve. Not until I lost my wellbeing did I realize I didn't want what I was achieving. I had lost my path and never thought to get back on it.

At heart, I am a free-loving hippie. I love to dress up with a dress-down edge. I love dancing, learning, teaching, big belly laughs, reading, trying new things, traveling, cooking, and drinking. I have a loud laugh and love big hair. That's me, when I peel away all the layers.

Trying to be someone I was not deep down inside did not feel good. It was as if I was pretending to be someone else each day. Put a smile on your face and pretend you are happy, put on the right outfit, arrange your desk just so—all so no one ever realizes how overwhelmed you are. It made me bitter, resentful, and rather mean, especially to those who didn't work as hard as I did at being someone else. It wasn't pretty, it wasn't fair, but that's what it was.

Some people find it easy to connect to what they value and desire. That wasn't the case for me. After feeling completely depleted by my life, I had to find a way to prioritize my actions so I could start actively engaging in life again.

My life lost all personal meaning. While that may be okay with a cashmere sweater, it's not okay in creating a life worth living. By being thoughtful, I stopped patterns that, over the years, had developed into habits that limited me. I was able create new ways of thinking and doing. That's why I am so driven to share how to Live with Passion, Purpose, and Play, in hopes of helping pave the way for you to create a Flight Plan that empowers you to create a life worth living. Without Thoughtfulness, there can be no meaningful connection to what you desire, and you will get the same results you have always gotten in your life.

Before you can reclaim your time, you must be clear about how your day-to-day actions will contribute to your success. To get this clarity, we must look at what you want, what is going on in your life, and what has happened. Following are questions to gauge your feelings, thoughts, emotions, and motivations.

Moving Forward – Teresa

Teresa is a very successful nutritionist and health coach. She is not married and has no children. She helps people every day get on a path that supports their health using diet and exercise. She loves her business, and since it took off so quickly, she hadn't thought about how she wanted to grow personally or professionally. When she called me to help, she wanted to find ways to work more efficiently and update her systems.

Teresa managed a very successful business for five years. During that time, she took on more clients than she should have, considering her obligations and responsibilities. When she started making mistakes, feeling sick, and letting people down, it was time to do something about it.

In working with Teresa to create her Flight Plan, we looked at what she wanted her days to feel like, what types of things she enjoyed doing and wanted to do more of, what she wasn't enjoying anymore and wanted to do less of, what she could do to feel more of what she wanted and less of what she didn't, and how she wanted to work and with whom. The results were mind-blowing for her, as she realized how much of her time was wasted because she wasn't thoughtful of what she wanted for herself. She had flown by the seat of her pants since her business took off. She hadn't looked back or thought of what she wanted to do next for herself or her business.

Through working her Flight Plan, Teresa has discovered what she wants now and where she must invest her time to get the desired results. She has reclaimed control of her time and her dreams. After a year, she has more digital products and fewer clients, which has allowed her more time to enjoy long breaks to travel and care for her needs. Teresa relies on her Keys to achieve success by her terms, and she revisits her terms regularly so she doesn't forget what she is working for.

Where Are You Now

If you want to gain clarity and wisdom, you must reflect on where you have been and what you have gone through. Answer the following questions to learn more about your character. Take as much time as you need. Use this exercise when you feel lost and don't know essential information about yourself.

What are your hopes and dreams for your future?
What are your personal strengths and weaknesses?
What are your passions?
What are your beliefs?
What are your values?
What is your philosophy about life?
What have been your proudest accomplishments?
What have been your perceived failures, what
caused them, and what would you do differently
if you had the same experiences again?
How do you see yourself?
How do you want to be seen?
How do you see the people who have
significant roles in your life?

While doing this exercise, I realized I had never looked back or brought light to any of my issues and problems. I had simply locked them away in the pit of my belly. I realized that several characteristics of my personality did not reflect who I want to be or how I want to show up in the world. So, I made a conscious decision to notice my positive and negative traits and behaviors. These questions helped me discover my likes and dislikes, my strengths and weaknesses, and my overall character.

When I was blessed with another chance at life, I craved reinvention. I wanted to slow down, make things more effortless, and feel again. I wanted to create an authentic, heart-centered life for myself. I poured over the characteristics I had developed and made part of my personality over the years. I modified and, in some cases, completely extracted all characteristics I felt would keep me from achieving the character I knew would best serve me as I recreated myself from the inside out.

By developing a heightened sense of thoughtfulness, we can give more of ourselves to others, which results in stronger relationships and greater confidence and self-esteem. It is time we take personal responsibility for how our personalities, emotions, and behaviors can affect us and those around us.

Let's put pen to paper and answer the questions above. Make a conscious decision to be more thoughtful with yourself and others.

The problem is not that the Material World gives us too much. The problem is that we don't know what to do with what it gives. We don't know how to take what is of service to us and leave the rest behind. We don't know what we want. We don't know how we want to live. We don't know how we want to be known. We don't know how we want to feel. We don't know what we don't know.

Explore! Decide what you want, and when the Material Worlds gives you another option, ask yourself, "Will this help me?" If so, take it and infuse it into your day-to-day life. But if it doesn't, let it go. Drop it like a hot potato and get back to creating a life worth living.

Key 2 | Regulate

Do you ever regret not doing something?

From attending happy hours to watching movies and everything in between, we numb ourselves with activities we would happily give up for growth. It's happened to me more times than I care to count, which is why I have set up boundaries and triggers to remind me to behave in a way that I've decided supports me best in achieving my life's goals.

This Key requires we regulate what we do and what we allow into our lives.

My friends tell me they don't understand how I can live with so many rules, but that's not what these are. These are directives that keep me aligned with what I consciously choose for myself. They are controllers of how I want to be to achieve my goals, those things I truly and deeply crave. This is monumental, yet so many just don't seem to get it.

Being clear about what we truly desire is important, because when we're tired and stressed out, we don't think clearly about the things we truly desire. We think about what feels good immediately. The problem is that what feels good immediately may not, and often does not, feel good later.

If you've had a rough day at work, eating a double cheeseburger with mustard and a bag of fries with ketchup may sound like a good idea and feel good immediately. But later, when you start feeling sluggish and can't think, you chastise yourself for not choosing better, because that burger's giving you heartburn and keeping you from focusing on what you must do. These mini-dramas may play out with a different set of circumstances and cast of characters, but the results are always the same. You are no closer to where you want to be, and that doesn't feel good.

For me, food represented love, comfort, and recognition. It is everything I needed and didn't have the courage to ask for. It was the help I needed in the kitchen. It was the supportive friend that didn't judge me or reveal my secrets. It was everything life was not at the time.

How to Regulate

Regulating allows you to invest your time where you will gain the best and highest returns for your wellbeing. This will give you more opportunities to create ease and flow in your life so the experiences you have enhance your quality of life.

Create Boundaries with Ease

A boundary is a dividing line. Boundaries can be set around the things that don't support you in achieving your goals. Boundaries can also keep you from doing things that don't support what you want for yourself.

Creating boundaries is necessary to keep out what doesn't belong.

To Regulate, you must:

First, know what you want. I hope you understand by now that you *must* know what you want. The end game. The outcome. The deeply desired result. You must know how you want to feel and be willing to explore things that make you feel that way. It's not enough to know you want to be happy. You must first know what it feels like to be happy. Then, you will be led to what can make you happy. Be forewarned, it doesn't always "look" how you imagine, but it will feel better than you ever hoped.

I honor your desire to create the transformation you want to experience in your life, but reading this or any book will not help you unless you do the work. It took me two decades of reading personal development books to fully understand that. In the hundreds of self-help books I have read in my lifetime, none of them told me this. But it was what I desperately needed to hear, so I have to say it to you here.

Second, know what you have to do. Create a list of all the things that have to be true for you to achieve your goals and life dreams. These are your boundaries. This list is generated from all of the things you need and want to do each day, both personally and professionally, that support you in achieving your fullest potential and those feelings you desire. It can include grocery shopping, cleaning, cooking, taking a bath each night, journaling, meditation, saying affirmations, calling mom once a week, working late once a week, or creating a date night. It includes everything you want to do regularly to make sure you Live with Passion, Purpose and Play. This is the part that keeps you from sacrificing your health, wealth, and happiness while you are achieving success.

Third, create triggers. A trigger causes an event or situation to happen. When creating triggers, think of behaviors you can practice to give you the needed resources to do the things you want to do. Consider:

How do you want your days to flow?
When will you call those you love most to catch up?
When will you reach out to friends?
When will you schedule those getaways?
When will you go shopping, clean, and do groceries?

Using the list of boundaries that you've written and the way you live each day, think of behaviors and tasks you can execute every day to support what you want to create for yourself. Look at what you can group together.

Have patience as you take on new behaviors and functions. Ingrained behaviors and habitual tasks are difficult to change, so give yourself time to adjust. I don't want you to become overwhelmed and quit because you feel too much is going on.

Live by Your TERMS

When we give so much of our time and energy to others, we don't leave enough for what matters to us. Making the right decision for ourselves requires considering the cost of a YES. When contemplating a YES, we must consider the TERMS—the Time, Energy, Resources, Money, and Sanity.

During a high-level training at High-Performance Academy, my mentor Brendon Burchard introduced me to the concept of evaluating your TERMS. Here is my take on what it means to live by our own TERMS.

Time. Time is a commodity. When the clock stops, it stops, no matter what we are doing. We are only allotted a limited amount. When considering an opportunity, gauge how much time it will take and decide whether you have time available to invest.

Energy. If you know what it's like to lack energy to do the basics, you understand that energy must be highly regarded. If you commit to doing something, show up energized and enthusiastic. Otherwise, what's the point?

Resources. Considering what you are being asked to do or the opportunity being presented, ask yourself what resources you will need or have to create if you say yes.

Money. You absolutely must consider how much saying yes will cost you in dollars and cents. Dedicating funds to this opportunity may mean saying no to another one, so money and cost matter.

Sanity. Don't say yes to anything that will drive you nuts and that you won't enjoy. Always consider what else you want to do and have to do. Be honest about whether or not you have time to take on something else.

After evaluating the TERMS, measure your desire.

What is the reward of saying yes?
Is this something you really want to do?
How are you feeling about your decision?

In the end, it comes down to how you feel about the thought of saying yes or no. It is important that you say no to things you don't want so you can say yes to things you do want.

There are times when I look at the TERMS of an opportunity, and even though I don't get all of the answers I want, I still feel there is a reason I should do what I've been asked. Some things cannot be evaluated with logic, and we must go with our hearts. While these types of situations should be few, they exist and must not be ignored. What's critical is that you make a conscious decision.

Ease Into the "No"

Saying no and hearing or seeing the disappointment from the other end is not easy. Sometimes, what is being asked is simply inconvenient at the moment, and you may not really want to say no. In that case, offer an alternate solution. Understand that saying no does not mean you have to justify your decision. "No" is a complete sentence, but using it can be difficult. Instead of justifying your no, consider saying, "No. Sorry I can't make that work." You don't have to explain why. Have this simple statement as your go-to for saying no more easily, and, eventually, the "no" will come easier and with less guilt.

Key 3 | Assign

Assigning is transferring your tasks and triggers into your agenda to give them their due time. You will literally look at your day, with your list of what you want to get done in hand, to decide how and when you will take action. Assigning allows you to honor your boundaries so you don't feel overwhelmed and overloaded as you create a life worth living.

We all talk about how busy we are, but we don't talk about whether or not we are making ourselves busy with the things that really matter—the things that add true value to our lives. To live a life of meaning and connection, we must create meaning and connection.

Assigning helps you make the most of each and every day. Knowing what you want and practicing this Key will keep you from suffering through fire drills and last-minute rushes that leave you feeling overworked and unappreciated.

Ways to Assign

There are two effective ways to Assign. Both allow you to do more while working less.

1 | Delegate. As you review your list, consider delegating things you don't have to do yourself. Be creative and ask others for help. Remember, just because you can do it doesn't mean you should. Share the workload and responsibility by delegating tasks to someone who can do them at least 80% as well as you can.

2 | Schedule protected time to take inspired action. Be creative as you lay out your schedule. Keeping our lives organized keeps us out of overwhelm. Each and every day, renew your commitment to invest time to organize so you can enjoy more of what brings you happiness. From making time to enjoying lunch with your best friend to grocery shopping, give everything a place in your schedule. You will love the end result, which is never saying, "I wish I would have . . . " Life is too short to live with regrets so remember to plan for the fun stuff too.

Create an Agenda

Creating an agenda filled with what you want to do from day-to-day will give your days shape. Without direction, we tend to spend more time than we should thinking about what to do and investing too much of our time on a single task, while ignoring everything else we have to do to keep life running smoothly. Usually, we end up doing what is in front of us and not what matters to us. When you invest your time doing things you want to do without neglecting what matters, the quality of your life experiences takes on a whole new level of joy.

Build Your Schedule

Look at your calendar and create time to do the things that will allow you to live with Passion, Purpose, and Play.

What will you do to achieve and maintain a Thriving Mindset?
What will you do to Calm the CHAOS?
**How will you achieve the level of connection
you want to experience in your life?**
What will you do to have more health and wellness?
What are the first dreams you will make a reality?
**What day of the week will you organize
the next week for more ease?**

**When will you practice your spirituality,
and how will you do it?
How will you infuse Passion, Purpose, and Play into
your day so you can do what you need and want to
do faster and achieve the success you desire?**

When you look at your habits, ask yourself, "Are they making it easier or harder for me to support my desires?"

If they are making it easier, excellent. Keep on doing what you are doing.

If they are making it harder, take a step back. Reflect and identify what is out of alignment with your deepest desire to invest your time in creating a life worth living.

To create a Daily Agenda, fold a sheet of paper vertically into three equal sections. Title the left column "Daily To-Dos." In the second column, write the first twelve hours of the day in 30-minute increments, going down the page. In the third column, write the last twelve hours of the day in 30-minute increments down the page.

In the first section, Daily To-Dos, write the things you want to do each day.

Next, write and block the times in your schedule when you have to be somewhere. Include recurring daily appointments and your regular commitments, obligations, and responsibilities. Include things like meditating, exercising, reading, journaling, and anything else you want to make sure you do daily.

Next, look at your week and note specific things you want to do on specific days. Record those tasks on those days.

If you want to limit certain things during the week, find the best days on your schedule to make that happen. As an example, I limit my intake of animal products to three times a week. For me, that does not mean the same days each week. I look at my calendar and note days I will dine with others or go out for dinner, and I'll preplan to eat meat during those times, knowing I will be tempted.

It is important to be conscious of the way you want to live, and create the best environment to support you in the way you have deliberately decided you want to experience each day so you stop living by default and start living by design.

Your daily schedule should be filling up at this point. As you schedule your waking hours, you may feel like there is too much to do. Instead of getting stuck in overwhelm, there are a couple simple things you can do to reclaim your time.

How to Stop Overwhelm

Take a critical look at your to-do list.

Do you have to do everything on your list that day?

Get your tasks done each day in order of importance, not appearance. Tasks you don't need to do right away can be moved to another day that looks lighter.

Are there any deadline-driven projects on your to-do list?

Break these down into manageable tasks you can easily execute in one- to two-hour blocks, each taking you closer to completing your project on time without frustration and overwhelm. There is nothing worse than looking at your never-ending list of things to do only to realize one of them will take days instead of hours.

Everything in your life cannot hold priority status.

Things to do are the result of living. If you do run out of things to do, you know what that means, and no one wants that . . . right? At least, not until it's time.

Protect your time.

During your workday, prevent wasting time between tasks by transferring your tasks into your schedule and blocking time to take action. Literally, create an appointment to act. This is your protected time. Honor it. Never allow other people's emergencies to supersede what you have scheduled to do during this time.

Your agenda is what drives your days. Every day is an opportunity to experience the depth and meaning you crave, while creating a purpose-driven life. This is what will help you stop feeling as though you haven't accomplished anything when your head hits the pillow. When you live with purpose, your purpose gives you life.

My Agenda

As an example, I'll share what this looks like in my life. Following are my personal boundaries and triggers for creating a life worth living—as defined by and for me.

> Journal every day.
> Drink lemon ginger detox tea every day, the recipe follows.
> Detoxify each week with a coffee enema.
> Drink at least 1 green smoothie each day, the recipe follows
> Bust a sweat 6 days a week for at least 30 minutes.
> Meditate twice a day for 20 minutes each time.
> Drink 8 to 10 glasses of water each day.
> Pick up the house every other day for 1 hour.

Deep clean the house twice a month for 4 hours.

Eat solid foods 2 times a day.

Eat meat 3 times per week.

Take a 12-hour break from food each day.

Work standing up at least 4 hours of each work day.

Go for a long weekend at least twice per year.

Go on a family vacation at least 1 time a year.

Go on a romantic getaway at least twice each year.

Enjoy a romantic evening on the town at least 1 evening each month.

One day a week, relax, rejuvenate, and rejoice.

Sleep at least 7 hours but not more than 9 hours each day.

Read at least an hour a day.

Read 1 fun, purposeless book each month.

Reach out to at least 3 family members or friends each week.

Check in twice each day on my energy levels and if I am living up to My Words (see the Reflection in the Spiritual Prescription for Commitment for how to define your own).

Live with Passion, Purpose, and Play.

In creating my schedule, I thought about my days and when I like to work. Since I'm a morning person, I enjoy getting the bulk of my work completed by the early afternoon.

Every day starts much like this:

6 a.m. Trigger – Reminder set to "Awaken in gratitude and prepare for an amazing day." I set this as a reminder, not an alarm. I get up when I get up. However, I normally wake between 5:30 and 6 a.m. This trigger reminds me to give gratitude, prepare and drink my lemon ginger tea, meditate, and journal about how I feel and what I'm looking forward to.

As soon as I wake up, I give gratitude. I literally open my eyes and say "Thank You." I find waking up in gratitude enables me to take on the day with love rather than fear.

I drink three cups of water.

Then . . .

Mondays

Monday is coffee detox day. I prepare the mixture while I journal and look at my schedule for the week. I figure out the days when I will clean, grocery shop, and do laundry. I schedule my household work around my other scheduled activities for the week. Then I meditate. I drink lemon ginger tea after the coffee detox. I close this ritual with meditation and mantra. This takes 90 minutes.

8:00 a.m. to 9:30 a.m. I pay bills and prepare for my finance meeting with my husband.

9:30 a.m. to 11 a.m. Finance meeting with Fred. We use this time to discuss our finances, any special purchases we want to make, and report how our businesses are doing.

I do not normally work on Mondays unless I am traveling. The rest of the day, Fred and I spend time running errands, enjoying long lunches, laughing, and talking about what is going on in our lives.

I take a nap before I prepare dinner. Nap time is a new habit for me. I like to take 30 to 45 minutes to refresh. I don't get to do it every day, which is why it still feels like a luxurious experience. I never understood the value of napping until I started allowing myself to enjoy this mid-day break.

Once a month, we make it a point to stay home to deep clean the house. During this time, I also do laundry for the week.

Tuesday through Friday

I start my lemon ginger detox tea. I journal while I wait for the ginger to steep. I continue writing while I drink my tea. Then I meditate. This process is about an hour. Then I start working.

8 a.m. I prepare a smoothie and get back to work as I drink it.

In the mornings, I am a force to be reckoned with. I am ready, willing, and able to get through anything. During this time, I am alert and make excellent choices and hence practice these rituals, which help me show up for my family, my friends, my clients, and myself.

I work out from 30 to 60 minutes.

11 a.m. Check emails, specifically for those I'm waiting on.

12 p.m. Trigger to check in with My Words. Each day, I want to show up loving, passionate, and present. I have an alarm that reminds me this is how I want to be. This also reminds me to check my schedule so I stay on task.

12:30 p.m. Alarm to stop for a lunch break. On Wednesdays and Fridays, I stop my work day here, if possible. This gives me time for a nap, meal planning, cleaning, and laundry.

2:15 p.m. Alarm for trigger asking, "Is this the best use of my time?" I also check my energy levels and respond to emails.

4 p.m. Alarm to start wrapping up the work day. I check where I am and what still needs to be done. During this time, I usually take

a breather with a cup of tea and a book for an hour. Then I prepare dinner and dine with my family. Meal time is usually around 6 p.m.

7 p.m. I check and respond to emails from my private clients. What I do after dinner depends on my workload and my need for relaxation and fun.

8:30 p.m. Reminder for Me Time. No matter the workload or what is going on, I do something I enjoy and that makes me happy.

9:30 p.m. Trigger – Rest Well, Beautiful Soul. This is my trigger to prepare for bedtime. This means taking care of my personal needs, reflecting, and journaling about my day.

Saturday

I start my lemon ginger detox tea. I journal while I wait for the ginger to steep. I continue writing while I drink my tea. Then I meditate. This process is about an hour.

I work out from 30 to 60 minutes.

The rest of the day is my own. I invest the time organizing, cleaning, reading, doing laundry, and the other things I didn't get to during the week. If I am up to it, I go to the Farmer's Market or do some grocery shopping.

Once a month, I have breakfast or lunch with a good friend.

Sunday

Sundays are my favorite day of the week. In the early morning hours, I enjoy my detox tea, quiet reflection and relaxation, journaling, and meditation. This normally takes about two hours.

Depending on my needs, I'll either go grocery shopping in the morning or clean. For me, cleaning is like detoxing. The process feels energizing.

After 10 a.m., the day is dedicated to enjoying time with my family. I may prepare brunch, go out with the kids, or have everyone over for a family dinner.

The evening consists of more relaxation and watching television with my hubby.

I hope this helps you see how I use all the information I gathered from asking myself the same questions I posed to you. I fill my days with the actions that will lead me to the experiences I want to create for myself.

Be flexible and check in often to confirm you are living with Passion, Purpose, and Play by investing the time to do the things that will make the difference between surviving and thriving.

Recipes

Following are recipes for my lemon water ginger detox tea and smoothies, in case you were interested in trying them. For the coffee enema detox mixture, Google "Gerson Coffee Enema."

Recipe for Lemon Ginger Detox Tea

½ cup filtered spring water – room temperature
½ cup filtered spring water – hot
½ organic lemon
2 nickel-sized slices of fresh organic ginger root
Dash of organic cayenne pepper

Boil a ½ cup of water. While the water is boiling, cut and dice your ginger. Remove boiling water from the burner. Place the ginger in a teacup and pour in the boiling water. Let sit uncovered for 4 minutes. Then add the room-temperature water to the ginger water and add the lemon juice. Finally, add a dash of cayenne pepper.

Recipe for Simple Smoothies

I keep my smoothies very simple.

> Place 1 cup of low-fat Greek Yogurt/organic coconut water/coconut milk/almond milk/rice milk in a blender with:
> 2 cups of power greens (blend of spinach, kale, and baby greens)
> 1 apple or ½ apple and ½ banana
> 3 ribs of celery
> 3 carrots
> 1 heaping teaspoon of organic, high quality matcha green tea powder
> 1 cup of frozen fruit

Blend and drink.

* * *

Okay, deep breath. I know this is a lot and, for some, too much. Please don't feel your day has to look the same. I have been conditioning myself for the last seven years to live with this full schedule. I want and enjoy a full schedule. That's me.

I implore you to create a life worth living by using what I've shared to define what that means to you and for your days.

Key 4 | Vigilance

This Key is about taking focused action. Singular focus is how you can do what you have to do with more ease and faster.

Completing the tasks on your calendar and setting the intention to do things when it's time is half the battle. Too often, we are easily distracted by one thing or another. From our email inbox to our social media, everyone wants to tell us what to do with our time.

Think about what has happened over the last week—occasions when someone or something distracted you from doing something you needed or wanted to do. Think of how you could have eliminated that distraction. It could be as easy as placing a sign on your office door, saying "Working on Important Project, Please Do Not Disturb," or allowing your voicemail to take a message and calling your friend after you've completed the tasks on your calendar.

Every time you switch gears, ask yourself, "Is this the best use of my time right now?" If the answer is no, stop and do what you feel would be a good use of your time. Remember, control the flow of your day and make it fun. This is what fulfills your joy and brings you happiness.

A word of caution here . . . Be flexible. Do what feels good and right for you. Again, I am not talking about short-term gratification. I am talking about what you will be happy doing five or ten years from now. Will it feel good in ten years to know that you finished school? Took the time to mend a fractured relationship? That you finished that big project? Moved to another state? This is how you assume the responsibility for your wellbeing.

Some days, you may decide to give yourself a break when you have already scheduled your day. If you have given yourself ample time and taking a break now will not cause overwhelm later, go for it. If you struggle with focus, following are a few ways to maintain your momentum and inspiration to do what you have to do.

Focus on What You Have To Do

Work during your best time.

Some of us are morning people. Others hit their stride in the middle of the afternoon. Identify your best time of the day; this is when you get down to more complicated business. Take care of your detailed and complex work when you feel most energized and engaged. Save returning phone calls and emails for times when you are looking for simple work to complete.

Turn off your notifications.

We all get distracted by the dings and beeps coming from our devices. If you have trouble ignoring them, turn them off. Just because someone texts, calls, or emails you doesn't mean you have to answer immediately.

In conversation after conversation, I hear what a time suck and energy waster social media and email are for many. Some feel guilty for enjoying it. What I recommend is scheduling time to check your emails and socialize on your favorite social media platform, and stick to it. If you enjoy being on Facebook, give yourself permission to spend a certain amount of time on it each day by scheduling it into your agenda. Then stop beating yourself up. How you spend your time is your business, and if it makes you feel good, you should wholeheartedly enjoy it—without guilt and stress.

Do only one task at a time.

Getting sucked into multitasking is easy, and many of us believe we do it well. However, if you look back to the times you felt most overwhelmed, were they when you were working on three things at once? I'm guessing the answer is yes. This is definitely true in my experience.

Studies done by Professor Earl Miller, a neuroscientist at the Massachusetts Institute of Technology, have revealed that those who multitask are up to 40% less productive than those who do not.

We have discussed how to say no more often, but this is a good time to mention this again. We often give too much of ourselves and waste time with things that we don't want to do, either by taking on other people's problems or overextending ourselves. Again, say no to what you don't want so you are available to say yes to what you do what.

Create a Capture Place.

Oftentimes, as you focus on one thing, something else pops into your mind. You can use a notebook for this. If you prefer to work digitally, use Evernote or a similar application or program. While working on other tasks, as things or thoughts come up that you don't have time to address at the moment but want to remember, record them in your Capture Place.

At the end of the day, take 15 minutes to do those things that will take five minutes or less each. If you write a note to watch a movie or read a book, move it to the appropriate list; if you intend to do it in the near future, put it in your schedule. Then assign, or schedule, the remaining items so you can take action when you have time available to invest. This will help you make the most of your time, energy, and days.

Do what you say you are going to do when you say you are going to do it. Let nothing distract you or keep you from doing the things you are fully committed to achieving.

Key 5 | Extract

Let's look at things that may be slowing you down or blocking you from achieving the goals you have consciously set for yourself. Do you know what these are?

They are those piles of papers, magazines, and bills on your desk or the floor of your bedroom, the exhaustive lists of things to do that leave you feeling overwhelmed, or your digital inbox overflowing with emails and photos.

This Key is about taking care of those piles, real and virtual, by creating processes and systems so you can effectively manage everything as you receive it.

"Everything" includes:

> Your Paper and Electronic Mail;
> Incoming Calls and Voicemail;
> Text Messages;
> Magazines and Newspapers; and
> Whatever else you want to add to this list that is unique to your lifestyle.

A Spiritual Girl creates systems and processes to keep the piles and her days under control. Otherwise, the chaos takes over, and she doesn't feel like she's moving ahead with clarity.

Information comes at us from all directions. By creating a simple way to examine and extract what we need then expel the rest, we will feel calmer and more settled knowing we're not missing anything that matters.

Go through your paper and digital information to extract what you need and want. Here's a system you can use. You may have seen it before. I have been using it for many years. I am not sure where I learned it first, but since that time, I have read and heard it from many sources.

4-Step System to Evaluating Everything and Extracting What Matters

Step 1 | File. Classify your digital and paper information the same way. If the information you decide to file is related to auto insurance, label your file "Insurance | Auto." If the documents relate to home insurance, label your file "Insurance | Home." Keep your filing system simple and be consistent. If you over-complicate this part of the process, you will get frustrated when you want to locate your information.

Step 2 | Action. Take action at first interaction. If something you receive can be handled by someone else, assign the task out immediately and schedule a follow-up date so you don't forget about it. If you can take care of the issue yourself in five minutes or less, and you have time, go ahead and take immediate action.

Step 3 | Schedule. If a task will take more than five minutes to complete, look at your schedule and place it on your to-do list for that day so you can take action when it's convenient. You will feel less stress this way. Plan an extra 12 to 15 minutes per hour in your workday to take care of small, less time-consuming tasks and unplanned emergencies.

If you have a particularly busy lifestyle, don't schedule more than three hours of your work day with things you must absolutely do. Inevitably, things will come up, and you want to create a buffer to deal with the unexpected issues that arise. This will allow you to do what you want to do and need to do without going into overwhelm or feeling frustrated.

Step 4 | Toss. If you receive garbage, real or virtual, throw it away. When you receive information that is not useful for you, don't pile it up. Throw it out! If you put something aside, schedule time to review it.

Create Lists that Make a Difference

No doubt, there are tons of lists that lend themselves to the chaos and confusion of what to do next. Creating lists for the sake of creating lists can feel overwhelming. Yes, you need to get things into an organized, well thought-out list, but typically, this means having one huge, overwhelming list that keeps you feeling frustrated and stuck because you don't know where to begin.

Once upon a time, a long, long time ago, I had many sleepless nights, remembering all of the things I didn't do that day and what needed to be done tomorrow. By morning, I would forget the majority of my mental lists and would sit drinking my coffee, frustrated and overwhelmed, wondering, "What was it again I need to get done before I leave for work, or get done at lunch, or what running around do I have to do after work?" Have you ever been there?

After years of practice, I am now the queen of meaningful lists. I know what I want to do, what I need to do, and when it needs to get done. It has given me peace of mind and freedom to enjoy life as it comes.

Top 10 List of Lists for Effective Productivity

Lists 1 through 4 | Daily, Weekly, Monthly, and Annual Lists.
Know what you want and need to accomplish each and every day, week, month, and year. Add any time increments unique to your lifestyle, like quarterly or semi-annual lists.

List 5 | Someday List. Write out a list of projects you want to complete. Go ahead and dream a little about what you want to do for yourself and those you love.

List 6 | Book List. Keep a running log of books you want to read.

List 7 | Movie List. Keep a running log of films you want to see. Also, create a sub-list of your favorite movies. Think of it as creating a playlist of music, except instead of music, the list contains movies that move you in the emotional direction you crave.

List 8 | Play Time List. If you're anything like me, when you get a moment for play, you don't know what to do. I created a list, and when I have a gap in my schedule that allows for some play, I immediately go to my list and plan a little adventure to suit my mood. This list helps.

List 9 | We Time List. With life moving us faster than we like, at times we disconnect from family and friends we enjoy. Keep a list of people you want to connect with regularly. For some, this may seem needless. However, busyness often keeps us from thinking of or getting in touch with the people we love as often as we would like. This list means never saying, "It has been too long," to someone you care about but have become disconnected from.

List 10 | Me Time List. Showing ourselves a little love doesn't always come easily, and we certainly don't think of it as often as we should.

Make a list of things you can do to care for your needs, even when you only have 10 or 15 minutes. This will make it easy to decide quickly, without much effort, what you can do to put more pep in your step.

I write my daily, weekly, monthly, semi-annual, and annual lists on index cards. This makes putting what I must get done in my Flight Plan much easier. I refer to these index cards to get started. Then I add to the index cards the tasks I need to complete to get me closer to accomplishing one to three projects that are on my Someday List.

I keep my Book, Movie, Play Time, We Time, and Me Time Lists digital, so I can access them anytime.

Keep lists of books to read, documentaries to watch, places to travel, and any other category that interests you. If you write these down, it is more likely you will read, watch, and travel, as you desire. Commit to doing one thing on your list each month. Schedule which month you will take inspired action and set up a reminder. This will help you stop feeling like you are missing out and saying, "I've been wanting to do that," or "I've always wanted to go there."

Emptying your head of all these details means being able to do what you want and need to do without missing a beat, making you a miracle worker without the "work."

From which piles, real or virtual, can you extract what you need and want?

Go through your piles, taking time to quickly review everything and put each item in one of the four categories: File, Action, Schedule, or Toss.

253

Plan a day to go through them now. If a whole day freaks you out, schedule a few one-hour sessions and see how far you get.

By taking this simple action, those piles will not only be gone, but they will be dealt with in a manner that honors you and the way you want to live.

Key 6 | Learn

This Key focuses on learning for your personal and professional development. Be open to learning new things to bridge the gap between fear and faith. Many of us have certain expectations of what our days should look like, though they may never happen due to changing circumstances or conditions. What's imperative is that we embrace change and be open to it. This is where this Key comes in.

Improve Yourself

This is an opportunity to get to know yourself on a deep level. I have been exploring my inner self for several years and am finally reaching clarity on what I want my life to mean at this stage. I feel as if I have been on a sojourn, learning to define my life purpose because it means different things at different times. Even as I make this statement, I know there is more to come. There is for everyone.

Here are a few questions that will help you gain clarity and give you what you need to practice this Key.

Am I happy?
What do I want to have, be, and do?
How can I get what I want?
What is keeping me from having what I want?

If you are unsure about the answers to these questions, they will come in time. As you live with Passion, Purpose, and Play, you will continue clearing your way so you can gain clarity.

Improve Your Systems

If you notice inefficiency, solve it. Find your bottlenecks and tighten up your systems as you go. Replace what doesn't work or what doesn't work as well as it used to. There is no need to re-create the wheel or re-vamp all your systems at once. As you move throughout your day, ask yourself if you are doing things the fastest and best way possible. We get stuck just doing, not wanting to force ourselves to try something new. It's essential that you work as efficiently as you possibly can. Doing so means doing what you have to do faster, saving you energy and time.

Many people do things the way they have always done them because that's the way they learned to do them. They do this even when they know there's a better way. This is why it's not only important to learn but to use your knowledge to make things better than they are now, even when they are already good.

Improve Your Tools

Learn how to utilize technology to save time and help you work efficiently. Too often, we buy things that overwhelm us, constantly saying, "I don't know how to do anything on this phone but talk," or "These devices are so hard for me to understand. I just use it to watch movies."

Before we spend our money on the latest and greatest gadget, we need to ask ourselves, "Why am I buying this?" If you have valid reasons and decide to make the purchase, take it one step farther and commit to learning how to do all the things you listed in your reasons to buy.

For Growth

Learn the things that will move you further in your life. Focus on a learning challenge every 30 days.

What has really helped me grow is focusing on a topic and getting to know more about it. Over the last few years, I've been obsessed with business and spirituality (I know, what a combo). One month, my challenge will be to learn everything I can about landing pages, then the next month it would be to learn about Archangel Michael. I'm a multi-passionate so you just never know what will move me next. What's important is you choose to learn about what interests you and moves you forward. If you come across something you want to know more about, create 30-day challenges for yourself on topics that interest you. Create a Growth List based on the following questions:

What can I learn to improve myself?
What can I learn to improve my tools?
What can I learn to improve my systems?

Select the things you read and watch according to these lists. This will help you achieve more while doing what you enjoy.

Commit to making one of the things from each of these lists happen each month. Depending on how much time you have available to create more meaning and happiness.

Key 7 | Self-Love

I believe this is the most worthwhile Key, and it's a reminder to always to be kind to yourself and be your greatest fan.

Too many people lose connection with who they are and what they want because they don't make themselves a priority. This includes not honoring their desires or needs, speaking poorly of themselves, and allowing others to dim their light.

We all do it. We say we are the priority in our lives, but at the end of the day, we put our needs last on our list. That's not in alignment with creating a life worth living, is it?

In the 30 or so years before I experienced The Illness, I felt I needed to do everything and be everything for the people in my life. It was not only necessary for me to show up, but I also wanted everything to be perfect.

Then I broke and was stuck in bed, unable to keep my closets organized, my baseboards and fans dusted, my pantry organized with all labels facing forward and fully stocked with our favorite family foods, or the laundry done just so. It took years for me to realize the perfection I was trying to attain was an illusion.

We must stop wasting precious time trying to attain perfection, taking control of everything just because we think we can, and doing things we really don't want to do. We must create time for the things that fill our happiness meter. We need to make happiness investments with Me Time, We Time, and Play Time. I hope you are ready to fully embrace this idea and give yourself a break, because you deserve it.

Create Your Self-Love List

Take a few deep breaths to quiet your mind. Tune In and explore these questions.

What does self-love mean to you?

How could you show yourself more love?

Then, make a list of 50 things you enjoy doing now and enjoyed as a child.

Finally, go back and circle 25 of the things that appeal most to you.

If you are struggling to create your list, check out Mr. Googs (Google) and search for "fun ideas for adults," or phone a few friends and ask them what they do for fun.

Happitunities

Me Time, We Time, and Play Time fill our happiness meter. I call them Happitunities. These are the ways we invest our time that help us get off A path and get on THE path to living with Passion, Purpose, and Play.

Schedule Time for Happitunities

Each day, we have things we must do for our survival. Scheduling Happitunities as one of those will reenergize your mind, body, and soul so you can experience life's successes. No matter how much success you create in the Material World, if you don't take the time to enjoy the journey, your wellbeing will suffer, and you will not realize the good stuff you worked so hard to achieve. I implore you to make yourself the priority.

Me Time

Block out time to do the things that make you feel good. Take a long bath, read a book, go for a relaxing dinner, or jumpstart your wellbeing with a sojourn. You are the most important person in your life, so treat yourself that way.

This is one of the more difficult time commitments for us to embrace because we don't give ourselves permission to treat ourselves well. If you have trouble making a commitment to Me Time, just think how much better you would feel after giving yourself time to clear your head and how that would affect your relationships.

The consequences for not taking at least 15 minutes a day for yourself can be devastating. If you get sick, who will take care of everything?

Bestow Admiration for Yourself

Admiration is about developing a deep love and respect for yourself.

Show yourself love.
Respect your body and fulfill your energy.
Declare your admiration for the amazing Spiritual Girl that you are.

Gratification

Gratification is about pleasure, especially when gained from the satisfaction of achieving a desired goal or state of mind.

Allow pleasure into your day.
Invite it in with a special treat.
Fulfill your energy by spending time with those you love.
Declare your gratitude for the amazing, beautiful soul that you are.

We Time

As I shared when I spoke about Connections earlier, strong social ties are critical to our emotional fitness. We are talking about people you love being around, people who fill you up. You feel good when you are around these people, and you trust they have your best interests at heart.

Play Time

Play is a journey rather than a destination. The experience of play makes us happier, healthier, wealthier people. By allowing guilt-free, purposeless play into our lives, we are better able to connect on a meaningful level with ourselves and others, and handle the stress that living in the Material World brings with it.

We tend to dismiss play for adults because it is perceived as unproductive, petty or, at its worst, a guilty pleasure.

Play is meant to be purposeless, voluntary, fun, and pleasurable.

Think art, books, comedy, cooking, daydreaming, flirting, movies, music, and traveling. It's all play.

It's time to rethink play and infuse it into your every day.

Play Time is important for all aspects of your life, so it's time to give yourself permission to act like a goofball, pull silly pranks in the office and at home, or create time to read a book with an entertaining story. Surround yourself with funny people and bring on the good times more often.

While we want to infuse play throughout our day, we also want to schedule dedicated Play Time.

If you start to feel Play Time is a guilty pleasure or a waste of your time, remember the incredible benefits you and your family experience because of your enlightened attitude.

Be Creative

Rather than your typical outing with your love, family, and friends, get creative. Go to a theme park, paint, or go on a scavenger hunt.

Join a food stroll or go to the park for a walk. Do the things you normally do on vacation but in your home city.

The Reflection Process

Openly and honestly answer the following questions weekly to keep you on your path to creating a life you love. I block two hours on Sunday mornings to do my reflection. Choose a good time for you to reflect each week. Set a reminder and honor yourself by doing this work.

What were my highs?
What were my lows?
What did I do well and enjoy? What did I do well and wish I could do more? What did I do well and wish I could do less? What did I not do as well as I hoped? What did I not do well and wish I could? What did I not do well and never want to do again? What did I feel passionate about? What made my heart sing? What made me smile? How did I deal with people, events, issues, challenges? Did my actions this week represent how I want to be seen?

Review what you wrote.

How does it make you feel?
Are you happy with your responses?
Is there anything you can do today, tomorrow, or in the future to live a life that will make you more comfortable with the responses to these questions?

Do not judge yourself. Just give attention to your physical sensations and emotional being as you respond.

Doing this work is what creates the clarity in what you do, where you go, and what you say and to whom from day to day.

By learning from what you don't want to experience, you can bring into your life exactly what you want. This contrast helps you develop clarity. The more clarity you have about how you want your life to look and how you want to feel each day, the more deliberate and directive you can be with your time and energy. The momentum you build in transforming the way you experience the Material World will absolutely delight you in every sense of the word.

Be Selfish with Your Self-Love

Be selfish enough to schedule self-love. Block out one hour in three weeks of every month, and three hours in the fourth week for a self-love session. Schedule what you will do during each of these self-love sessions. Give yourself permission to do anything you want to do. Honor this time and do what fulfills you. Meditate, read, or pamper yourself. Have coffee or lunch or call a good friend. Take up a new hobby. Anything you feel inspired to do with this time is good for you. Practicing this Key will jumpstart transforming the way you experience your life.

* * *

The Keys empower you to live in alignment with your Passion and Purpose. They also keep you on task so you can do what you need and want to do faster, not so you can do more, but so you can Play more.

Each day, you can apply The Keys to keep you on path.

The Secret Key

Sometimes the Material World's chaos takes on crazy momentum, and you just want to run away. Far, far away.

It's not a bad idea. In fact, it's a great one.

I'm not saying forever. I am saying consider taking a real break from your demands, obligations, and responsibilities. It's a lot and can weigh heavily, especially when you are worn out and stressed out.

The secret key is TRAVELS. You may have picked up on it since the 7 Keys to Thriving Productivity are:

Thoughtfulness
Regulate
Assign
Vigilance
Extract
Learn
Self-Love

TRAVELS

Have you ever noticed how many travel
magazines are in your doctor's office?

These travel magazines connected me to special times in a way that surprised me.

They reminded me of when Fred and I went away for our anniversary every year for over a decade. We loved Las Vegas. It held special meaning for us. That's where we honeymooned, and each trip always reignited our passion and brought us closer. We occasionally went to

Mexico, but it was usually Las Vegas; we didn't experiment much or go off the beaten path. That's just who we are.

The magazines reminded me of family times as a child when my mom and Abuellos took me to Puerto Rico. That's when I saw my mom at her strongest. We visited family and went to the beach. I went camping with my grandparents. These times created some of the most amazing memories that I still cherish today.

They reminded me of fun times when my bestie Cindy and I took our kids away for fun weekends, while our husbands worked. We let our hair down and explored new areas with our children. My daughter still talks about those trips.

During The Illness, I reflected on my life, as I'm sure most people do when they are going through a similar time, feeling helpless, hopeless, and losing faith. As I looked back on some of my favorite times, I realized they were when I was traveling, experiencing the essence of the Material World. The memories and bonds created during those expansions carried me through some rough times and helped me when I needed it most.

No matter how you travel, you have to admit it changes your behavior and challenges you to reflect on where you are in your life. Think about it. It's really the only time we allow ourselves to decompress, do some soul searching, do the things that bring us joy, and consider where we are.

As it turns out, this is not an accident. It is the result of our physiological system recovering from the noise and chaos of the Material World.

The Benefits

According to the U.S. Travel Association, taking vacations can improve health in several measurable ways.

An annual vacation can cut a person's risk of heart attack by 50%. Blood pressure, heart rate, and levels of epinephrine decline on holidays within one or two days. As a result, we sleep and feel better.

At least four out of ten travelers feel more romantic on vacation, and nearly one-third admit to making love more often on vacation.

When you vacation, there is a 25% to 50% increase in performance after returning. Three out of four executives believe that leaves are necessary for them to prevent burnout or that vacations improve their personal job performance. Two out of three believe vacations enhance their creativity.

According to Dr. Mel Borins, author of *Go Away Just for the Health of It*, for every $1 saved by employees not using their vacation time $7 is lost to health care and lost time from people not being in the office or not being productive.

What I'm sharing with you here is just the tip of the iceberg. There are hundreds of benefits to traveling.

In my recovery, when I thought about what I wanted to do about work, I knew I did not want to return to the confines of another law office. Office politics really wore me down, and I wanted nothing to do with it.

I clung more and more to these reminiscences of travel because of the amazing experiences and the beautiful memories, and I decided to go into travel when I was ready to return to work.

In 2012, I started my travel business. I focused on customized Wellbeing Getaways set up to support growth and healing. Because of my experience with isolation during The Illness, I wanted to help people during challenging times to think differently.

I send groups of four and up to 200 on transformational journeys that I called sojourns. Before the trip, I sent each traveler a series of emails that helped them get ready, so they didn't feel stressed out preparing to leave. These emails included bonding ideas so those going on the trip could start the connection process before they went away together.

I was overwhelmed with appreciation by what was reported to me. My clients often told me the first thing they shared with others about their trip was my email series. They loved it. They are the ones who encouraged me to start speaking and writing a blog. From there, my career as the Wellbeing Messenger took off and led to me writing this book.

Wellbeing Travel

The trips I plan are not ordinary journeys. I customize the travel so it is not the kind of vacation you feel you need another vacation to recover from afterwards. They allow for growth experiences and healing. I've studied, at great lengths, how the body is affected during and after travel, how the body and mind rejuvenates, and how to make the most of the time away.

Too many people binge when they vacation. They "treat" themselves. They play full out every day. As a result, they return home more exhausted than when they left. The euphoria of their vacation wears off quickly, and they never truly get the actual benefits of a vacation.

Most of us don't take proper advantage of our time away. This happens for a couple of reasons. The first is some vacationers don't get away enough, so when they do, they go all out and whoop it up. The second is, while some vacationers get away, they don't fully disconnect from the weight of their obligations and responsibilities. Finally, for some, since they are so used to living in chaos, they don't know what to do when it is not present. Thus, they cause drama and sabotage their experiences.

The 7-Day Wellbeing Vacation Experience

There is a special recipe to the perfect vacation. By "perfect" I mean one that includes what you must have to calm the chaos, reclaim your time, and transform the way you experience the world.

Relax First

Flying is stressful for your body. The long lines, getting through security, and the process of flying create anxiety and tension. It doesn't make sense to put ourselves through that since the point of going away is to detox from the stress. But there's not much we can do about the process. Since we are aware that this happens, let's plan to take care of it.

The first day you arrive at your destination, rest. Rest four hours for every hour you flew. This first day is ideal for exploring your hotel or the resort where you're staying, laying out by the pool or on the beach, a spa treatment, eating healthy food, and indulging in things that bring you comfort and, more importantly, that keep you relaxed.

Have an Adventure

On the second day and fifth day, do something fun and exciting, something you are enthusiastic about experiencing. Take an excursion and explore your environment. Sign up to do something you have never done, which challenges you to open your mind.

> **The 2012 U.S. Travel Survey conducted by the U.S. Travel Association revealed that when you are on vacation, you naturally bond with those you do fun things with, whether they traveled there with you or not.**

Isn't that awesome? Again, one of the many perks of travel.

Love Yourself

On the third day and sixth day, treat yourself to a spa experience to rub out tension and toxins from your body. Plan on a fun-filled evening, perhaps dancing and a culinary experience. Nothing speaks to the soul like good food and spirits.

Go Explore

On the fourth day, get to know where you are. Immerse yourself in the local culture. Travel like a local, visit the local shops, and get to know the people of your destination.

Go Home

On the seventh day, go home. Allow for relaxation, reflection, rejuvenation, and rejoice in the good times you just had. Too often, we get caught up in life as soon as we return home and forget to relish the incredible experience we just had.

If you don't have time for a seven-day vacation, start your vacation by focusing on what you need first. If you have more than seven days for a vacation, lengthen the time you allow for each activity.

Get Away

Now it's your turn. Go away. Go far, far away.

Plan a getaway for yourself, but do so mindfully by thinking through what you want to go away to achieve.

Choose Your Companions

Tune in to how you are feeling and why you want or need a break. Are you overcoming some personal or health issues? Are you too stressed and need to get out of town before you explode or implode? Who do you want to be surrounded by while you are enjoying your time away?

By choosing travel companions who share common interests and are easy to talk to, you guarantee a spectacular vacation. When you decide on your travel companions, plan a dinner or small gathering to test run the group. You want everyone to get along and mesh well.

There is nothing worse than trying to bring together people who, quite frankly, just don't get along or don't jive with one another. It's like going through an awkward dinner party for seven days. Excruciating. Don't do it. Surely, that's one thing we have learned from all of those Housewives reality shows. (Yes. I confess. I'm a fan of all the Housewives shows.)

There is no absolute, right number for how many people you want to share a long weekend or vacation with. However, I find everything and everyone works well in pairs and quads for getaways. It's hard for someone to feel left out when everyone has a partner. I recommend traveling in fours: four, eight, or twelve, for individual getaways. For couples, typically four to six couples.

Decide on a Budget

Traveling with a similar idea of a budget in mind ensures a harmonious getaway. Definitely discuss this in advance with your travel companions. Budget affects virtually everything you do, where you stay, what you eat, and how you get there.

Choose a Destination

The destination for your vacation should be fitting to your needs and desires. Be sure to consider any physical limitations you or one of your travel companions has.

Put Your Vacation on the Calendar

Make yourself priority number one and schedule your vacation sooner rather than later. Ideally, the date will be no less than three weeks and not more six months away.

Plan Your Entertainment

The plan is essential to a successful vacation. The time it takes to organize and plan the kind of vacation you want, need, and deserve is often underestimated. On average, it takes travelers seven to eleven hours to plan a vacation. Think about what you and your companions are interested in and like to do. Taking into consideration how you feel (physically and emotionally), make sure you plan something you and your companions will enjoy and take part in.

Make sure everyone's needs and desires are addressed in a way that will benefit the entire travel experience.

* * *

Ideally, we would lead lives from which we don't need a break, but this isn't the case. Travel helps us broaden our perspective and grow in ways we could not in our home environment.

Whether you can take four days or 40 days for travel, make the most of your time by doing the things that will help heal your body, mind, and soul.

Section 3

ARE YOU READY TO THRIVE?

Now that you know where you are, where you want to go, and how to get there, it's time to commit.

Commit to your health so you don't become a statistic.

Commit to your wealth so you don't get everything you want but are missing everything you need to create a well-lived life.

Commit to your happiness so you stop accepting surviving as the default for living a life well-lived and start thriving.

In Chapter 7, you will bust through the blocks and start living the life your soul intended by living your Flight Plan.

Chapter 7

Commit to a Life Worth Living

"Most of the important things in the world have been accomplished by people who have kept on trying where there seemed to be no hope at all." ~Dale Carnegie

You have finally reached the part of the book where I tell you that, because you know without a doubt who you are and what you want for yourself, you will live with more ease and peace than you ever thought possible.

But I can't do that. I hate it when people say things that aren't true just because they sound good, so I won't do that to you.

What I can tell you is this: Because you are awakened to what is possible, when you stray off THE path, the path you consciously placed yourself on, you will realize it sooner than you ever have before, preventing you from straying too far for too long.

I have been walking this more enlightened, spiritual path, choosing love over fear and using my emotions as my guidance system, for over seven years, yet, I still falter. There are still times when I don't trust my intuition and when I don't ask myself the questions I know will lead me to doing what feels and is right for me. But, because I am aware, when I check in, I quickly realize where I am and I get myself back on track. Because of this, I live in alignment more often than not, and you will too.

Knowing what you know doesn't mean you can let your guard down. I live in the light with fleeting moments of darkness. Because of my deep work, the work you are doing, I know in every moment I can choose again, and so can you.

Just when you think you've got it, someone or something will knock you off your path so far that you won't know if you will ever find it again. When that happens, check in. Come back. Recommit to creating a life worth living. Redefine what that means for you. There are no mistakes when modifying and enhancing your vision. Each day provides you with more clarity to create a life experience filled with joy and meaning.

When you fall on your face, pick yourself up, dust yourself off, and start all over again. Only when you refuse to learn from your experiences do you fail. No one has ever achieved anything great by refusing to try again, and again, and again.

Bust through the Blocks

It's important that you meet The Others where they are. They are simply reflecting their beliefs and experiences. They are not living consciously, looking at the Material World through eyes of love. They have not done the deep work, yet . . . They have not clearly and consciously defined what they want and who they are. They still live in the chaos of the Material World and have not mastered the beauty of it. They have not learned to utilize the chaos for the good it could do for them.

It is futile to share your new, awakened attitude and try to control what The Others think. As you model and enjoy a life you love, they will come around and ask what you are doing and how they can do the same.

That is when it is time to share what you have and are experiencing with every new waking moment.

Moving Forward

It is natural for new things to come up as you move forward and grow. I use a few rules to keep me on my path. When I start to feel nostalgic, and not in a good way, these rules keep me in my consciously chosen path.

Never Be the Victim

Things happens. Don't allow your life circumstances and the things you have had to deal with and overcome keep you from bringing the joy to your life. You are not defined by the situation you are born into or find yourself in.

When you slip into self-pity, focus on and appreciate what you have learned because of your circumstances and experiences. Never, ever beat yourself up about what was.

Never Live in Your History

Live in the present moment, focused on what is now. Don't go backward and replay your history for anything other than to learn from the experience. When you live in the past, you cannot move forward. You must give yourself permission to release the past that keeps you weighed down and keeps you from experiencing what you truly want.

Never Compare

As you move forward, it is easy to think about what could have been if you were on a more conscious path a decade or two ago. Understand and accept that that was not to be your experience. It if was, it would have been. Where you are now is where you are supposed to be. Never doubt that.

I have given into victimhood, history, and comparison more times that I care to count. No one is immune. What is important is that you recognize when you fall into the trap. Take yourself out by sitting back and reflecting so you can course-correct.

My months in bed were a blessing I did not recognize when it happened. It gave me perspective to determine what creating a life worth living means to me. It was taking those first steps, being aware, being willing, and being committed, that helped me get out of that bed and create this amazing, beautiful life I am blessed to live today.

Take the time you need to disconnect from the chaos, even if only for an hour each day to define what a life worth living means to you so you can create it, consciously. Stop going through your days only answering to the expectations of The Others and not creating any for yourself.

Living in the unconsciousness of the beautiful chaos of the Material World keeps us stuck and from experiencing all the phenomenal things it has to offer.

You now hold The Keys. You know what to do. You know how to get unstuck and move forward. You know, step-by-step, how to create the life your soul intended. The power is yours and yours alone.

Perfection is the Illusion

Creating a life worth living is not about striving for perfection. There is no such thing when it comes to living a conscious life.

We get caught up in thinking *if only this*, or *if only that, then . . . Only then, everything will be what I want it to be.* But time and time again, we have been fooled because when this or that happens, there is still something else that keeps everything from being "perfect."

Think about how boring life would be if everything was perfect. How would you grow with perfection? There would be nothing to strive for. There would be nothing to challenge you. There would be no learning or expansion in your life.

Granted, from time to time, we want to slow things down. Now that you know how to achieve a Thriving Mindset, Calm the CHAOS, and Reclaim Your Time by living with Passion, Purpose, and Play, you can execute your Flight Plan and do exactly that.

All you need to do is take a step back and a few deep breaths and start again. You can do this. We all can. Everyone is born with the ability to create a life worth living, but we lose our way. We get caught up in beliefs and experiences that stop us, but that's not you. Not anymore.

You know how to focus. You know what you want. You know how to use the beautiful chaos of the Material World for your best and highest use so you can show up as the loving, beautiful soul that you are and have always been.

All you must do is commit. And when you lose your way, commit again. Commit to creating a life you love over and over again. Until it sticks. Until it is uncompromising. Until it is in your subconscious.

You have all the tools you need. You know what it means to live with Passion, Purpose, and Play. You know health, wealth, and happiness are yours to be had and are your birthright. When you feel yourself stray, come back to the fundamentals. You have Spiritual Prescriptions to heal what ails your soul so you never feel lost or stuck again.

Have patience with yourself. Being a Spiritual Girl in a Material World takes practice and dedication. This is not something you do once. You do this over and over again. As you grow and evolve, the things you desire will change as well. Be prepared as you give yourself permission to allow this growth to come into your life. Don't fear it. Have the courage to face it head-on. The fear will hold you back and keep you from living a life worth living.

This Is the Time

Don't be someone who knows what to do but doesn't do it. I read and re-read self-help books for decades before I took action, and I delayed creating health, wealth, and happiness.

I believe I experienced the things I did because I did not take action on the lessons I was learning, so they kept playing out for me. I was stuck, achieving but not enjoying my success. About every ten years, I would have to step away from my life, change my friends, and change my home. Luckily, I didn't change my husband. I have someone who stands beside me no matter what I am going through and, while I didn't know it at the time, he is one of the biggest blessings in my life.

Someone once asked me to consider what my life would be like now if, at the age of twenty-five, I had the knowledge I have today. Where would I be? What would I have done differently? What would be different?

It wasn't necessary for me to wait until my forties to experience a life filled with Passion, Purpose, and Play. I was responsible for settling for where I was, wanting things to change but doing nothing differently, giving away my personal power to stop what I didn't want. But, as I have said, we are each on our own path. I am where I am supposed to be. For that, I have no doubt or regrets. I am where I am now because this is meant to be my legacy. I have taken all the lemons in my life and made the most delicious lemonade. And now, it's your turn.

If not now, when?

If not you, who?

You can continue to hand over your personal power and the responsibility of your health, wealth, and happiness to The Others. You can keep buying into the notion that you don't have a choice and that you have to blend in, because being different means standing out.

There is so much chaos in the Material World at this time. Truth be told, it scares me. I see millions of people lost in the darkness, and while I have the know-how and confidence to be of service, I can't bring people to the fountain of health, wealth, and happiness and make them drink. They must want it for themselves.

That brings us to my big questions for you.

Is it your time?
Do you want this now?
Are you ready to welcome health, wealth,
and happiness into your life?
Are you ready, willing, and able to create a life worth living?

Ready

If you are questioning your preparedness, rest assured that I know you're ready—because you are here. You raised your hand and identified yourself as a seeker. Whether you realize it or not, a part of you was awakened enough to pick up this book. That's enough to know you are ready.

Willing

I know you are willing, because you are doing the work: reading, thinking, processing; doing the exercises, digging deep, developing yourself so you can focus on what makes you feel good; willing to question not only yourself but everything around you.

Able

I know you are able because you have read this far. You are defining what creating a life worth living means to you. You have the tools, everything you need to do, step-by-step, to achieve all that you desire.

This is Your Time

Through your work in this book, you are recognizing what Living with Passion, Purpose, and Play mean to you.

Look how far you have come. You are giving yourself the gift of clarity of what you truly desire, as defined by you, without the noise and chaos of the Material World. You are defining how you want to live and show up in the Material World, and you now know how to do it step-by-step. This clarity allows you to live consciously.

You are laying out your path, and you know your destination with an image and vision you did not have before, so it is your time to take action.

Soar

You have everything you need to transform the way you experience your world. You don't have to wait until Monday, or for a new year, to live up to your full potential. You owe it to yourself to live your best life.

What you want will constantly evolve, and it is supposed to. As you gain new experiences, your vision for what is possible will grow. Embrace the process. Continue thinking of your life in terms of who you want to be and how you want to feel, then take the steps to make your dreams your reality. Always seek to reconcile your behavior with the lifestyle you want to achieve.

Even though the mindset lessons were the last part of what I truly understood as I recovered from The Illness, I shared them with you first for a reason. Slipping into old patterns quickly when I was stressed landed me in that bed in the first place, so I want you to have the mindset tools to identify and manage your patterns from the beginning.

Start Living

A Spiritual Girl lives in complete alignment with her beliefs, desires, and values. Life does not happen to her. She does not live by default, taking what comes her way and never asking for more. She takes action each day, with commitment and dedication to what she wants to feel. She is open to life's experiences without judgment or shame so she can acquire wisdom to fulfill her destiny and live the way her soul intends, honoring her feelings and trusting her intuition to guide her to her final destination.

Live your Flight Plan each day to become that Spiritual Girl. Begin creating a life you love by starting to live with Passion. Your mindset is critical to your ability to conceive what is possible for you. Next, focus on living with Purpose by defining what matters to you most. Finally, bring together your Flight Plan by living with Play and infusing the things that are most important to you to feel successful as you create a life worth living.

Start living the life you know is yours to be had. Don't let this be another one of those books you read, that you know can help you have and feel what you want, but that you put back on the shelf. Stop hiding your dreams in the shadows of your mind. Bring them to the light, and know that anything you desire is possible for you.

It is time to turn your dreams into your reality, and I've got your back every step of the way. I send you off into the Material World ready, willing, and able to create a life worth living.

In love and light, Beautiful Soul.

Take care of you and live with Passion, Purpose, and Play.

MEET THE AUTHOR

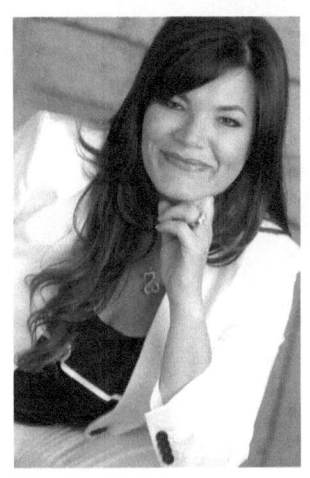

Carmen Perez is the founder of Wellbeing Messenger and www.WellbeingMessenger.com. She is a highly sought-after personal business success mentor and motivational trainer.

Carmen was blessed to receive a gift of illness – a second opportunity to create a life worth living – after surviving a battle with neurological Lyme disease that left her dismayed, depressed, and disabled. Since then, she has dedicated her life to helping people create a life worth living filled with passion, purpose and play. She founded Wellbeing Messenger for those who are tired of accepting surviving as the default for a well-lived life and are ready to succeed without sacrificing their health, wealth, and happiness.

Carmen inspires over 300,000 women a year through her blog, newsletters, products, and appearances. She has appeared on Fox News, Love Mexico, Wellbeing Travel Symposium, and television shows, podcasts, and other events with leaders and legends. Recognized as a thought leader, Carmen uses her wellbeing expertise to collaborate with tourism boards, hotels, and resorts to create consumer awareness and exclusive wellbeing travel experiences and packages.

She also motivates thousands of professionals and entrepreneurs from around the globe who attend her talks and seminars. Carmen's most popular seminars include *Get Noticed Online Now, Do More: Better and Faster, Create a Life Worth Living, and Create a Business Your Life Loves.*

Meet Carmen and receive free expert training at WellbeingMessenger.com.